What Readers Are Saying…

"Finally a book that gets at the heart of one of the most serious obstacles for quitting among women! Dr. Pomerleau knows her stuff after years of working with women smokers, and she shares the secrets to success in *Life After Cigarettes*. Don't miss the chance to make this book part of your quit plan."

— K., Ypsilanti, Michigan

"Good job…. I enjoyed reading it."

— L., Austen, Texas

"I really like the style—it's very warm and informative…. The list of resources at the end of the book is full of good leads."

— A., Milan, Michigan

"What I think is so great about the book is that it underscores the importance of post-cessation weight gain (and body image in general) as a *real* deterrent to quitting smoking. Women no longer need to feel that these kinds of concerns are unimportant or merely vain—especially since those are the very things that keep them from quitting."

— R., Mebane, North Carolina

"*Life After Cigarettes* is an inspirational book about learning to take care of yourself with a primary focus on quitting smoking. I am proud to say that I have made the choice to quit and even though I don't smoke anymore, this book has encouraged me to reevaluate my own exercise and eating regimens."

— R., Ann Arbor, Michigan

Ordering
Trade bookstores in the U.S. and Canada please contact:

Publishers Group West
1700 Fourth Street, Berkeley CA 94710
Phone: (800) 788-3123   Fax: (800) 351-5073

Hunter House books are available at bulk discounts for textbook
course adoptions; to qualifying community, health-care,
and government organizations; and for special promotions
and fund-raising. For details please contact:

Special Sales Department
Hunter House Inc., PO Box 2914, Alameda CA 94501-0914
Phone: (510) 865-5282   Fax: (510) 865-4295
E-mail: ordering@hunterhouse.com

Individuals can order our books from most bookstores,
by calling **(800) 266-5592**, or from our website at
www.hunterhouse.com

LIFE AFTER CIGARETTES

Why Women Smoke AND How to Quit, Look Great and Manage Your Weight

CYNTHIA S. POMERLEAU, PhD

Hunter House
PUBLISHERS

For further information please contact:

Hunter House Inc., Publishers
PO Box 2914
Alameda CA 94501-0914

Library of Congress Cataloging-in-Publication Data
Pomerleau, Cynthia Stodola.
Life after cigarettes : why women smoke and how to quit, look great
and manage your weight / Cynthia S. Pomerleau.
    p.   cm.
Includes bibliographical references and index.
ISBN 978-0-89793-525-8 (pbk.)
1. Women—Tobacco use.   2. Smoking cessation.   3. Women—
Health and hygiene.   4. Tobacco use.   5. Smoking.   I. Title.
HV5746.P66 2009
616.86'50082—dc22   2009024786

Project Credits

Cover Design: Brian Dittmar Graphic Design
Book Production: John McKercher   Editor: Alexandra Mummery
Copy Editor: Amy Bauman   Editorial Intern: Ashley Zeal
Proofreader: John David Marion   Publicity Associate: Sean Harvey
Indexer: Nancy D. Peterson   Administrator: Theresa Nelson
Rights Coordinator: Candace Groskreutz
Customer Service Manager: Christina Sverdrup
Order Fulfillment: Washul Lakdhon
Senior Marketing Associate: Reina Santana
Computer Support: Peter Eichelberger
Publisher: Kiran S. Rana

Printed and bound by Bang Printing, Brainerd, Minnesota
Manufactured in the United States of America

9 8 7 6 5 4 3 2 1   First Edition   09 10 11 12 13

Contents

IMPORTANT NOTE

The material in this book is intended to provide a review of information regarding smoking cessation, weight management, and mood modulation. Every effort has been made to provide accurate and dependable information. The contents of this book have been compiled through professional research and in consultation with medical and mental-health professionals. Health-care professionals, however, have differing opinions, and advances in medical and scientific research are made very quickly, so some of the information may become outdated.

Therefore, the publisher, authors, and editors, as well as the professionals quoted in the book, cannot be held responsible for any error, omission, or dated material. The authors and publisher assume no responsibility for any outcome of applying the information in this book in a program of self-care or under the care of a licensed practitioner. If you have questions concerning your nutrition or diet, or about the application of the information described in this book, consult a qualified health-care professional.

Foreword

The path that leads to a "Life After Cigarettes" is a circuitous one that brings women even more fully into touch with their bodies, albeit often in very uncomfortable ways. For many women, smoking is a friend, always there during times of stress and joy to smooth out the moment. And as nefarious tobacco companies have suggested to women for more than half a century, the thinnest women are smokers.

Does smoking even out mood through a learned pattern of responses or because of some biological cascade of events? Is the very real association between smoking and weight a result of substituting a smoke for a spoon? Or is there something in tobacco that burns calories in ways that rival some of the best FDA-approved weight loss medications? Perhaps even more important than mood and weight regulation, however, is the repetitive use of tobacco that has killed hundreds of thousands of women, and is the reason lung cancer deaths in women remain elevated even as lung cancer deaths in men have taken a downward turn. Is it habit, biological addiction, or some combination?

As Dr. Cynthia S. Pomerleau has demonstrated in her long career as a scientist dedicated to understanding the dynamics of smoking cessation, we are long past the time of thinking that tobacco use is just a habit; it is a biological addiction that requires immense personal strength as well as the best of modern medicine to overcome. But Dr. Pomerleau has shown that the challenges are even greater for women than for men. Relinquishing an addictive drug that also suppresses body weight and enhances mood, with the expectation of a broad spectrum of unpleasant withdrawal symptoms, is never easy. But for women who feel insecure about their appearance or not in control of their lives, it can seem close to impossible.

The book you are holding in your hand is the unique vision of Dr. Pomerleau. Having devoted much of her professional life to research on tobacco use among women, she was determined to share her findings directly with the many women smokers who are deterred from quitting by the fear of gaining weight, who worry that they can quit only at the price of feeling miserable about themselves and their bodies. She also wished to reach out to women who have succeeded in quitting but continue to struggle with their weight.

As Dr. Pomerleau points out, there are no magic bullets, no preset plans, and no certainty of the outcome when traversing the path towards a "Life After Cigarettes," but the good news is that there are many exceptional guides along the way. Dr. Pomerleau is among the very best! *Life After Cigarettes* offers new hope for women—not by providing a series of one-size-fits-all, step-by-step instructions for quitting and for controlling weight, but rather by giving each woman tools to develop the confidence and life skills she will need to become and remain, in Dr. Pomerleau's words, "a nonsmoker who feels good and looks great."

— Scott Leischow, PhD

Professor, Colleges of Medicine and Public Health, University of Arizona
Associate Director for Behavioral and Social Sciences Research,
Arizona Cancer Center
Immediate Past President, Society for Research on Nicotine and Tobacco
Former Chief, Tobacco Control Research Branch,
Behavioral Research Program,
Division of Cancer Control and Population Sciences, National Cancer Institute
Former Senior Advisor for Tobacco Policy, Office of the Secretary,
Department of Health and Human Services

Acknowledgments

This book could not have been written without the contributions of many people and institutions. At the risk of some critical omissions, for which I sincerely apologize, I wish to single out the following as being greatly deserving of my thanks:

The staff of Hunter House, especially Barbara Moulton, Alex Mummery, and Kiran Rana, have been as responsive and interactive as one could hope and a pleasure to work with.

Former members of my staff and other colleagues who provided a critical reading of the draft manuscript include Rebecca Namenek Brouwer, Raphaela Finkenauer, Lori Jones, Scott Leischow, Ann Mehringer, and Karen Saules. Keleigh Lee, Tia Moody, Dyan Osborn, Linda Howe Steiger (friend extraordinaire), and Fred Steingold (friend, author, attorney) also read the manuscript and graciously provided feedback and advice on various aspects of the text.

Research cited in this book and conducted at the University of Michigan Nicotine Research Laboratory was funded by the National Heart, Lung, and Blood Institute, the Robert Wood Johnson Foundation, and the University of Michigan Institute for Research on Women and Gender. The conclusions drawn from this research, however, are the responsibility of my coauthors and myself, and not of the funding agencies.

I am deeply grateful to the University of Michigan Department of Psychiatry for enabling me to devote 20 percent of my time for six months to work on this project. Ellen McCarthy meticulously copyedited the manuscript prior to submission and provided other less-tangible help and support as well.

My daughters, Julie and Aimée Pomerleau, and Julie's husband, Jeff Stafford, all read the manuscript and should be added to the list of lay readers above. In addition, they helped to create a supportive environment for this project and cheered me on with their enthusiasm. My adorable grandchildren, Augie and Claudia, provided welcome diversion along the way.

My husband, Ovide Pomerleau, my partner in work and in life, has been enabling and encouraging beyond measure of my work in general and of this project in particular. I could not wish for more.

Introduction

This book is for you if you want to quit smoking BUT...

* You gained twenty or thirty pounds, maybe even more, the last time you tried to quit.

* It is nearly spring, and you can't face trying on bathing suits if you gain even one more ounce.

* You fear your spouse's or your partner's put-downs, or even rejection, if you gain even a little weight.

* You became so depressed the last time that you stopped that you had to start smoking again after two days.

Or maybe you've already succeeded in giving up cigarettes, BUT...

* You can no longer squeeze into the clothes you used to wear.

* You avoid looking in the mirror while you're dressing.

* You still think longingly of the days when you could just light up when you felt blue.

* You wish there were some way to go back and "get it right."

If any of these comments sounds like your own thought process, then think again...and read on. This book is not intended as a stop-smoking book, or a cookbook, or a diet book, or an exercise manual—though you may find some useful ideas in all these areas, as well as a list of additional resources following the text. You won't be asked to fill out daily food diaries or smoking logs, or to follow a series of step-by-step instructions for changing your smoking or eating habits. Rather, this book is about personal style, regaining control of your life, and letting go of smoking and the comforts it provides by finding other ways to feel good physically and feel good about yourself emotionally. Above all, it is about looking terrific—in fact, better than ever before—when you're no longer smoking.

My conviction that this is possible is based on a career in research on smoking spanning more than two decades, much of which has been focused on women's smoking and, in particular, on concerns about gaining weight as a barrier to quitting. My knowledge about the effects of smoking in women, and the difficulties they face in quitting, comes from studies funded by the National Institutes of Health, the Robert Wood Johnson Foundation, and the University of Michigan Institute for Research on Women and Gender, and carried out at the University of Michigan Nicotine Research Laboratory.

Truth in advertising: I was never a smoker myself. Well, at least not like the smokers I saw every day in the lab. During my first year in college, I made such a concerted effort to become a smoker that I may actually be a former smoker as defined by the Centers for Disease Control and Prevention—that is, having smoked at least one hundred cigarettes in my life. But like Bill Clinton and his experiences with marijuana, I never succeeded in learning to inhale. Eventually, I concluded that periodic uncontrollable coughing fits weren't part of the sexy and seductive image I was hoping to cultivate and gave up trying. Only later did I come to realize how fortunate I was.

But over the years, I have worked with, given questionnaires to, and otherwise interacted with hundreds if not thousands of women smokers who were not so fortunate—asking them not only about smoking but also about their appearance and how they felt about themselves. One of the things that dawned on me early on is that the approach advocated by many of my mostly male colleagues—namely, telling women that the health benefits of quitting outweigh the health and cosmetic impact of gaining a few pounds—doesn't work. This is partly because many women gain more than just a few pounds and know this from their own past experience in trying to quit. But it is mainly because the issue isn't just physical health, and it isn't just health versus vanity. It is about how you feel about yourself, about the confidence with which you face the world.

Face it: There are definitely some plusses about smoking. If there weren't, you wouldn't have done it, and neither would anyone else. Then, once you're hooked, stopping causes a few days of intense longing for a cigarette, accompanied by mood swings and a sense that you're not on top of your game. Even after the initial intense symptoms of withdrawal subside, you may continue for months or even years to experience a desire to smoke and a feeling that something is missing from your life. It is just plain easier to keep on smoking.

Harder to see, and to hold onto in the course of day-to-day existence, are the plusses of *not* smoking. You're undoubtedly already aware of the long-term benefits of quitting smoking in terms of your own health and that of those around you. My goal in this book is to convince you of two additional things:

1. Some of the short-term plusses of smoking aren't what they're cracked up to be. Hollywood and Madison Avenue have sold us all a bill of goods—and smokers have paid the highest price. Although smoking suppresses weight and appetite, its overall impact on how you look and feel is detrimental—not just because of counter-advertising and social pressure that conspire to make you feel bad about yourself for smoking, but because of direct short-term effects of inhaled tobacco smoke.

2. Other short-term benefits of smoking can be achieved by alternative means—means that are more positive and self-affirming, means that will help you regain control over your own destiny.

HOW THIS BOOK IS ORGANIZED

The book starts with a discussion of why you smoke. It then explains how you can manage your weight during and after quitting, addresses special complications, offers help to those who are still struggling with quitting, and, finally, celebrates the joys of being a nonsmoker. At the end of the book, I offer my personal list of additional resources to keep you on the right track to managing weight and feeling great.

The beginning chapters frame the issues and provide background that will help in understanding the rest of the book. We've come a long way—in the wrong direction. How did we get into this mess? As Chapter 1 explains, the effects of nicotine happen to be well matched with the perceptions and needs of many women, and the tobacco industry has done its best to make sure we don't forget it. What the tobacco industry *doesn't* tell you is how smoking affects many other aspects of your appearance and body image—all unfavorably. Chapter 2 focuses on how body weight is regulated (the Energy In–Energy Out equation), and what happens when nicotine gets into (and out of) the act.

Chapters 3 to 5 are the heart and soul of *Life After Cigarettes*. Here, I share with you everything I've learned in more than twenty years of research about strategies to minimize the pain of weight gain, and how you can incorporate these strategies as easily and elegantly as possible into your non-smoking lifestyle. Chapter 3 covers the "Energy In" side of the equation and provides an approach to controlling your food intake, whether or not you choose to follow a formal diet plan. In Chapter 4, we move to the "Energy Out" side of the equation—how to incorporate exercise into your life and maybe even come to enjoy it. I also discuss the issue of what to do if you're *already* exercising a lot. Finally, in Chapter 5, we tackle the real, bedrock fear for many women—not just of gaining a few pounds but of having your weight spin out of control. This chapter tells you how you can keep your weight within your comfort zone and continue to look svelte regardless.

In Chapter 6, I address special concerns that may complicate your efforts. The first section covers relationship issues—how to handle a partner who is uncomfortable with your desire to change your eating patterns or a partner who is overly invested in your appearance. The second section deals with pregnancy and postpartum, times when the need to stop smoking and the need to control your weight may put you in a conflict situation. Some readers may need to turn right to the third section, which covers what to do if you are medically overweight or obese to begin with. The fourth section is about the minority of women who are threatened with weight gain in amounts that constitute a serious health risk. The fifth section explains how disordered eating patterns can seriously threaten your ability to manage your weight when you quit smoking. The topic of the last section is depression, which can undermine how you look by making you feel as though the weight of the world is on your shoulders—and on your midriff.

Although the focus of this book is on managing weight and mood without cigarettes, I recognize that some readers may still need help with the basics of quitting smoking. Chapter 7, "Quitting for Good," is for you. It provides a more detailed explanation of nicotine dependence, helps you identify the smoking cessation method best suited to your own "quitting style," and tells you how to find the support you need.

In the final chapter, I offer a lifetime perspective on becoming and remaining a nonsmoker. Chapter 8, "The Chic of Quitting," is about feeling good and looking great—the new nonsmoking you. Personal narratives of women who have struggled with concerns similar to those you're facing will help reassure you that you, too, can make it to the other shore.

Finally, at the end of the book, you'll find an annotated list of some of my favorite books, websites, videos, DVDs, and tools for weight and mood management.

I hope this book will motivate you to quit smoking, reinforce your commitment to staying quit, and serve as a companion as you say goodbye to this false friend. I hope you will visit my website at www.lifeaftercigarettes.com, where you can watch for updates and new ideas to help you succeed, gleaned from new research and from other women who, like you, want to quit and stay quit with style and grace. I hope you will send me reports of your triumphs (and even your failures) so that they can be used to help others. Most of all, I hope you will become *and remain* a nonsmoker who feels good and looks great.

What Every Woman Who Ever Smoked Should Know

There's something about women and cigarettes. The tobacco industry knows it, and so do you.

In October of 2002 my husband and I took a "*Carmen* tour" with a delightful English-speaking Belgian woman who—like the Pied Piper—led us and our fellow tourists through the streets of Seville, using an accordion and a backpack full of puppets and other props to bring to life the events in the opera. Carmen, the opera's fiery heroine, who may or may not have been a real person, was one of thousands of *cigarreras,* all of them women, who worked in the local tobacco factory. Men were banned because it was so hot in the factory that the women wore very little clothing. They often brought nursing infants in cradles that they rocked with their toes as they made cigars with their fingers—you can imagine the amount of nicotine those babies were exposed to!

The fascinating thing about these *cigarreras* is that they smoked while they worked, and what they smoked were cigarettes. That is not what they made in the factory, though, for at that time the factory was entirely devoted to the manufacture of cigars. It occurred to me then to wonder, "Was the cigarette invented by a woman?"

No historical evidence exists to support this speculation, so the question will have to remain unanswered. What can be said, however, is that women, at least in the Western world, have been amazingly loyal to the cigarette. While men have smoked cigars and pipes and used snuff in various forms, women (despite a few notable exceptions like Catherine the Great, for whom the cigar band was supposedly invented to protect her royal fingertips from tobacco stains, and Dolly Madison, who used snuff) have largely stuck with the cigarette. A remarkable current example is Sweden, where, possibly for the first time in the history of a Western country, substantially more women smoke than men, many of whom have switched to a smokeless tobacco product called *Snus*. Apparently, if there's nicotine in it, men will probably like it; we women are more particular.

Still, women's affair with the cigarette was not quite love at first sight. For much of its early history, the story of the cigarette is the story of men and smoking. Even after a Virginian named James Bonsack gave smoking an enormous boost in 1881 by inventing a cigarette-rolling machine that made mass production possible, and the advertising industry got into the act by developing and perfecting the concept of brand loyalty, smoking for women was severely stigmatized. Ladies were not invited to join men in "smoking rooms" after dinner, and they were barred from clubs and saloons where smoking flourished. In 1908 the Sullivan Smoking Act was passed in New York City, banning "unladylike smoking acts" in public places. Teachers caught smoking were dismissed on the spot; college women caught smoking were sent home. Only the boldest of women dared to smoke, and only the boldest of the bold ventured to do so in public.

Eventually, inevitably, the tobacco industry realized that women represented an enormous untapped market, and the campaign to normalize women's smoking began. It was abetted in 1913 by the development of the blended cigarette, a milder and better-tasting product that was easier to inhale. In 1919 the first ads targeted specifically to women appeared.

Up to this point, the spread of smoking among women followed a predictable enough course—going from being immoral and indecent to being naughty and daring to being widely tolerated, if not encouraged. But then something else took place. Smoking went beyond just being socially acceptable: It became a part of a woman's beauty kit and an instrument of personal charm. Smoking became a fashion statement. Smoking became chic.

How did this happen?

The answer, in part, is that the tobacco industry, the advertising industry, and manufacturers of tobacco-related products caught on to the fact that they could market the cigarette as something more than just a smoke. To get a sense of this "more," take a quick tour through the "Tobacciana" category on eBay. For several decades, there was (and, to a lesser extent, there still is) a brisk market in objects that framed the cigarette as a fashion accessory, as an article of makeup, as jewelry, as a component of a meal, and as an instrument for forming bonds of friendship and love. These products, along with other forms of advertising, had the effect of changing cultural beliefs about women and smoking, encouraging women and society to view cigarette smoking as not only acceptable but as highly desirable. (A similar process is now occurring in developing countries, with the predicted consequence that smoking among women worldwide will increase from its current rate of 12 percent to 20 percent in 2025. This change is already occurring in Turkey: Smoking, which used to be unacceptable for women, is now nearly as common among women as among men.)

I have been collecting women's cigarette paraphernalia for years, and among my possessions are a compact for storing powder, comb, lipstick, and…cigarettes; bejeweled cigarette holders and highly decorative cigarette cases (including one engraved with the words "I love you"); dainty folding ashtrays for travel; and souvenir cigarette boxes and lighters that serve as perpetual remembrances of honeymoons and cruises past. As for the connection with food, my collection includes luncheon plates with compartments for a sandwich, a cup of coffee, and…a built-in ashtray. I even have an ashtray in my china pattern! Sets of matching ashtrays meant to be used at bridge games and coffee klatches show that smoking together was part of the social glue.

Not just smoking artifacts but the cigarette itself became part of the "image." Articles in mass-circulation magazines of the 1930s and 1940s taught women the art and etiquette of smoking—how to hold a cigarette and how to exhale smoke in an appealing manner. In that era, 30 percent of women film stars smoked, and many actresses actually went to school to learn smoking-related body language—using smoking behavior to express anger, disbelief, and, of course, sexual attraction.

But as anyone who has ever tried to market tobacco substitutes quickly learned, even the cleverest advertising campaign could not have succeeded in creating such an aura around a product made with, say, lettuce leaves. Although for historical reasons, tobacco has until recently escaped regulation by the Food and Drug Administration (coming instead under the jurisdiction of the Bureau of Alcohol, Tobacco, and Firearms), tobacco contains nicotine—a potent drug. For starters, nicotine is highly addictive. This means that once you start smoking, for whatever reason and at whatever age, the "choice" to stop smoking quickly goes away for most smokers and quitting becomes a struggle, sometimes a lifelong struggle. Because nicotine is administered in frequent small doses accompanied by stimulation of all five senses, smoking becomes woven into the fabric of daily life in a way that is hard to disentangle.

In addition to being physiologically and psychologically addictive, nicotine has two properties that may make it especially seductive to women.

The first—and a central topic of this book—is its role as an appetite suppressant and tool for weight control. The tobacco companies were quick to catch on to the fact that this property of nicotine could be taken to the bank. In 1928 George Hill, an adman for the Lasker-Hill Agency, saw a heavy woman on a street corner chewing gum; soon after, he saw a svelte woman sitting in cab and puffing on a cigarette. "Eureka!" he said, and thus was born the slogan "Reach for a Lucky instead of a sweet." Later, threatened with a lawsuit by the candy industry, the manufacturer modified the slogan to "Reach for a Lucky instead…." But by then the damage was done, and almost everyone could finish the sentence without prompting. Just in case they couldn't, Lucky Strike launched a whole series of ads depicting a slim woman (or in some cases a man)—a swimmer, a diver, a horseback rider—backed by the shadow of a much stouter person. "Avoid that future shadow," the ads were captioned. "Reach for a Lucky instead."

Interestingly, the cult of slimness and the pressure to be thin date back to approximately this same period. The desire to be thin is not universal among women, either across cultures or over time. Indeed, in some eras and in some places, being a little *zaftig*—well-rounded—was a sign of prosperity and health. A plump wife bore witness to a man's ability to provide for his family. There are undoubtedly multiple reasons behind the aesthetic shift to a preference for thinness, including the development of mortality tables based on weight and height, the rise of movies as a source of standards for beauty and elegance, and the emergence of the carefree, boyish figure of the flapper. But it is also likely that the tobacco and advertising industries not only capitalized on this phenomenon but also contributed to it by making a virtue of the slimness their product promoted.

The second property of nicotine that makes it so responsive to women's needs is its association with depression. In both community surveys and studies of patients in treatment, smoking rates and amount of smoking are higher in individuals with depression. In other words, depressed people are more likely to smoke than people who are not depressed, and depressed people who do smoke are likely to smoke more heavily than nondepressed smokers. Although the reasons for this association are not well understood, there is some evidence to suggest that nicotine has antidepressant properties. It may also act indirectly by relieving stress. What's more, people who are depressed are more likely to experience depressed mood as a withdrawal symptom when they try to stop smoking. Not only does this undercut their chances of succeeding, it is also a serious quality-of-life issue that may deter many smokers from even *trying* to quit. Of course, this relationship applies to men as well as to women. But since the psychiatric diagnosis of depression is twice as common in women as in men, and since milder forms of depression, which affect much larger numbers, are also more common in women, the association of smoking with depression is particularly important for women. I wish I had a nickel for every e-mail we've received at the Nicotine Research Laboratory from women telling us they become depressed when they quit and asking where they can get help. A typical comment: "I don't want to go back to smoking, but I know the depression would go away if I did."

This is the discouraging dilemma that I referred to in the

introduction. Increasingly, however, women smokers and former smokers are looking for a way out of this trap.

Americans are at a tipping point in our thinking about smoking. More than ever before in recent history, we're ready to send this habit the way of the spittoon. Despite the sad and shocking persistence of smoking on the silver screen, it is an image many women no longer want to cultivate. For the first time in decades, fewer than one in five American women smokes. A recent *Monitoring the Future* survey found smoking among high-school students to be at its lowest rate since the survey began. Medicare recently made a long-overdue decision to cover smoking cessation treatment, signaling a growing recognition that smoking is not simply a "lifestyle choice" but a serious medical problem that cannot be solved by research on better methods for treating lung cancer. Nonsmoking is trendy!

You're probably reading this book because you want to be part of this trend, but you also need to resolve the discouraging dilemma produced by the persistent effects of stopping smoking on weight and mood. Smoking is sticky; there is no doubt about it. But based on my own research and that of others, I know that other women have succeeded, and so can you. I'm writing this book because I believe that with all my heart.

SMOKE AND MIRRORS

So who gains weight after stopping smoking? Sad to say, nearly everyone. Of all the documented tobacco withdrawal symptoms—anxiety, restlessness, difficulty concentrating, irritability, and so on—the most common one is weight gain. It is even more common than craving for cigarettes. Probably more than 90 percent of quitters gain at least some weight; for some people it is just a few pounds, for some it is much more than that.

Who cares? Many women do! My colleagues and I at the University of Michigan were fortunate to obtain funding for a national survey that included 371 daily and nondaily women smokers chosen at random from the phone book. When we asked these smokers how concerned they would be about gaining weight if they were to quit, about 40 percent answered, "Very concerned," which is consistent with other reports in the scientific literature. So if you have serious concerns about gaining weight if you quit smoking, you are not alone.

Does fear of gaining weight really deter women from quitting? Actually, women with strong weight concerns don't necessarily have more trouble quitting than women who are less concerned about weight—*once they've reached the point of enrolling in a formal treatment program*. The catch is that many women with serious concerns about gaining weight never even try to quit. We don't see them in our smoking cessation clinics because they stay away in droves. How do we know this? Admittedly, detecting something that doesn't happen is difficult, but remember the Sherlock Holmes story about the dog that didn't bark in the night, leading the detective to deduce that the intruder was not a stranger? Sometimes what doesn't happen should lead us to ask more questions.

One approach we used to investigate this issue was to study women who signed up for smoking cessation treatment but then failed to show up for their first session. We compared two different programs: One program targeted women with strong concerns about weight and body image, and the other program did not. The trials were similar in length and intensity of treatment. Sure enough, the number of women who dropped out before attending even one session was five times as high in the program aimed at women with strong weight concerns as in the other program, even though the women accepted into the other program happen to have smoked for longer, were more nicotine dependent, smoked more cigarettes per day, and had higher levels of depression—all factors that might be expected to make it more difficult for them to quit.

Another approach we adopted to determine whether or not weight concerns discourage women from trying to quit was to ask about both weight concerns and intentions to quit smoking in a national survey of women smokers. We found that women who had strong weight concerns expressed lower motivation to quit smoking and had less confidence that they would succeed in quitting if they tried than women who were less concerned about gaining weight.

This is something that many people—especially men—just don't get. Dr. Joseph Califano was the U.S. Secretary of Health, Education, and Welfare from 1977 to 1979, when public health campaigns to discourage smoking were getting into high gear. Later, looking back over his time in this office, he stated that if he had the chance to do it again he would have focused far more attention on the barrier to quitting posed by the fear of gaining weight. He went on to say, "Even though I gained thirty pounds in 1975 after [quitting], I did not appreciate the great importance to women of the link between quitting smoking and gaining weight." If we'd had a woman HEW Secretary at that time, and she had stopped smoking, I'm sure a thirty-pound weight gain would have grabbed her attention!

It is easy to trivialize this concern ("Why would anyone sacrifice her health to avoid gaining a few pounds?" or even worse, "How could anyone be so shallow as to sacrifice her health for the sake of her appearance?")—but it is also very unfair to do so. After all, a fact well known to behavioral psychologists is that small, immediate consequences are more powerful in influencing human behavior than consequences delayed by many years, even if these consequences are dire. Moreover, much of the weight gain happens early in the quit attempt—in some instances, several pounds within the first few days—just the time when smokers are hardest hit by the difficulties of breaking their addiction to tobacco and most vulnerable to temptations to resume smoking.

Remember too that we women, smokers or not, are socialized early and intensively to care about how we look—which in contemporary American society includes a strong emphasis on weight. It is easy to underestimate the power of this attitude and how deeply rooted it is. An evolutionary psychologist looking at what we've inherited from our prehistoric forebears might argue that, since men were physically stronger, women could only prevail by pleasing—and pleasing, as we know, is all too often bound up with appearance. For American women today, what pleases is thinness. Thin is in.

Finally, as we read in the papers and see on television on a daily basis, many people—even many smokers—are already overweight, often dangerously so. For obese women, weight gain is not just a cosmetic issue; it is also a serious medical concern. Attempts to downplay the dangers of weight gain compared to those of smoking, however well intended, are at best an oversimplification.

It is often believed, by the way, that weight concerns are primarily the white woman's province and are limited to countries and cultures in which thinness is prized. Indeed, when we first started to seek funding for our work on weight concerns among women smokers, I was criticized when I asserted that we were going to study women of all races. Weight control smoking, the reviewers argued, is a problem of white women; black women, they insisted, don't worry about their weight.

I eventually had an opportunity to test this belief in two different groups of smokers, one consisting of black and white women interviewed in a national telephone survey, the other of black and white women who had participated over the years in studies at the University of Michigan Nicotine Research Laboratory. Results from the telephone interviewees and the research volunteers were remarkably similar. The black women were several pounds heavier, on average, than the white women; their ideal weight was also several pounds heavier than that of the white women. The *difference* between what they actually weighed and what they wished to weigh, however, was almost exactly the same for the black and the white women.

In other words, the cutoff for acceptable weight was higher, on average, for black women, but the line is still there, just as it is for white women. Black women might use words like *firm* and *fit* rather than *slender* and *slim* to describe their preferred look, but it means as much to them as *slim* and *slender* do to white women. So although it may be correct to say that "thinness" is less valued by black women than by white women (again, on average), it is *not* correct to say that weight is not an issue for black women.

Bottom line: Most women, regardless of race and whether or not they smoke, would prefer not to gain weight; indeed, many would like to lose weight, and many need to lose weight according to the medical profession. So, women smokers are faced with a dilemma: They've heard all about the hazards of smoking, but they also know they are likely to gain weight. What's a poor smoker to do?

As the tobacco industry has reminded women in successive waves of advertising, nicotine has what most women would regard as a positive impact on their appearance—that is, it suppresses body weight. What the tobacco industry has neglected to mention is that smoking has many other effects on appearance and body image, and virtually all of these effects are negative. Many of these effects are a reflection of accelerated aging and of the antiestrogenic effects of smoking; note that women smokers tend to reach menopause a year or two earlier than nonsmokers. Other effects are the product of local irritation or effects on blood circulation.

The best known and most readily observable of these effects is on the *skin*, including increased wrinkling, crows' feet, lines around the eyes and mouth, age spots, enlarged pores, and dry, leathery-looking skin. Smoking releases an enzyme that breaks down collagen and elastic tissue. In addition, it can damage DNA, which may have a harmful effect on the skin. Smoking also reduces the amount of nutrients reaching the skin and impedes the removal of waste products from it. Wound healing is slower in smokers, with postsurgical infection and scarring (including recovery from cosmetic surgery and laser resurfacing) more likely.

A few years ago, Dr. Darrick Antell, a Manhattan plastic surgeon, made a splash in the media with a study he conducted on identical twins, in which he identified smoking as the skin's biggest enemy. Most shocking were the accompanying photos, in which the smoking twin consistently looked several years older. These twins are genetically identical, so the differences in their appearance are attributable solely to differences in environment and lifestyle.

In a 2004 interview, actress Susan Sarandon, age fifty-eight, when asked what she did to keep her youthful complexion, replied, "Well, first off, don't smoke…I do think smoking is really bad for you. I dabbled a bit when I was younger, but for most of my life I haven't smoked. And I do see the difference between people of my age who have smoked all their lives and those who haven't."

Here is a laundry list of the other negative effects smoking can have on one's physical appearance:

* Smoking has negative effects on *hair* and can lead to premature graying and hair loss.

* Smoking is associated with staining of *teeth*, and with loss of teeth due to the increased incidence of gum disease in smokers. Bleeding gums, receding gums, and a variety of other unsightly conditions are more frequently seen in smokers.

* Smoking stains your *fingertips* and causes cracked and discolored *fingernails*.

* Smoking can damage your *clothing*—think cigarette burns and more frequent washings to remove the odor of stale tobacco smoke.

* Smoking has negative effects on *posture and movement*. It contributes to osteoporosis—bone loss—which (in addition to increasing your risk of falls and broken bones) causes the so-called dowager's hump. It is also associated with rheumatoid arthritis, whose victims suffer joint stiffness and difficulty walking.

* Even the effects of smoking on weight are not unequivocally positive, since smoking affects *body shape* by producing changes in body fat distribution, probably due to its antiestrogenic effects. The waist of a smoker is larger in proportion to the size of her hips, on average, than the waist of a nonsmoker of comparable weight. In other words, women smokers tend to have less feminine

bodies—that is, less pear-shaped and more apple-shaped—than their nonsmoking counterparts.

In addition to changes in appearance, smoking affects other aspects of body image and physical attractiveness:

* Excess gum disease leads to more *halitosis*—bad breath—in smokers.

* Smokers on average have lower-pitched *voices* than age-matched nonsmokers, probably because of swelling of the vocal folds, the part of the vocal tract that vibrates when you speak and determines the pitch of your voice. Smokers' voices may also be hoarse and gravelly due to "smoker's cough" or polyps. (A colleague of mine said the clearing of her voice was one of the first things she noticed when she quit smoking—enough so that she felt inspired to join her temple choir after not having sung since high school.)

* Tobacco *odors* persistently cling to hair and clothing—not to mention your furniture, curtains, and other absorbent household surfaces.

* In menopausal women, smoking appears to exacerbate hot flashes.

These are not rare and unusual effects that may affect two smokers in a thousand, compared with one nonsmoker. These are common effects experienced by most smokers, effects that happen later, or not at all, to nonsmokers. If you're over thirty, you've probably noticed at least some of these effects already.

By now I hope I've convinced you that the effects of smoking on body weight are only a small part of the story. To the extent that your cigarettes have been part of your personal beauty regimen, it is time for a new idea.

There's nothing wrong with wanting to be the most attractive "you" you can be, and to have the sense of well-being that goes with looking and feeling good. In fact, there's a long and honorable tradition of caring about the impression you're making and recognizing that it makes a difference. The Italians call it "*fare bella figura*," roughly translated as "to put your best foot forward." Don't ever let anyone put you down or "dis" you for caring about your appearance.

The point is, smoking doesn't make you look better or more attractive—in fact, quite the opposite. There are far better ways to take charge of your weight and appearance. The sooner you internalize this conviction and begin to translate it into ways that work for *you*, the sooner you will become a successful former smoker. By successful, I mean not just a person who no longer smokes cigarettes, but one who has actively embraced her nonsmoking status and one who feels good about herself and her world. That's the goal, and you shouldn't have to settle for anything less.

2

Managing Your Weight and Looking Great: Making Friends with Mother Nature

The first step in reaching your goal of managing your weight and looking great as a nonsmoker is to get back on good terms with Mother Nature. Although you almost certainly didn't realize it at the time, your relationship with her started breaking down the day you started smoking. Tobacco—and more specifically nicotine—hijacks the mechanisms she so generously provided to protect you and keep you in harmony with yourself. Of course, there are many ways to get these mechanisms out of synch. Crash dieting, for example, can also do a pretty good job of it, and so can chronic overeating. But tobacco smoking is among the most treacherous, because it is so thoroughly woven into the fabric of your life. Think about it: By the time you've lived ten years as a pack-a-day smoker, you've taken nearly three-quarters of a million hits (or puffs). Twenty years: Double that. That's a lot of monkey wrenches in the works.

Fortunately, Mother Nature is forgiving. When you stop feeding the beast, she will welcome you back into her embrace.

Let's start with a brief review of nature's own plan for maintaining body weight and how nicotine (along with other aspects of modern life) disrupts these mechanisms. Your adult weight is essentially a function of "Energy In" and "Energy Out." "Energy In" is basically the calories you take in via food and drink. "Energy Out" consists of four components:

1. your basal metabolism—the energy your body expends just in keeping your cells, tissues, and organs alive while at rest

2. the energy required to digest food

3. the energy required to heat your body

4. the energy required for movement or physical activity

The first three of these are often lumped together as "resting metabolism"—the calories expended when you are completely inactive. Together, they account for about 75 percent of energy expenditure, with physical activity accounting for the remaining 25 percent.

Resting metabolic rate is lower in women than in men (but you already knew that, didn't you?). It decreases with age, so unless you moderate your diet over time you will gain weight as you grow older (the standard pattern for American adults), *whether or not you are a smoker.* Although this process occurs gradually over time, many women detect a noticeable jump in weight at menopause—probably the result of hormonal changes. Greater amounts of body fat, fasting, and crash dieting are associated with a lowered resting metabolic rate. Larger body size, greater amount of lean body mass, lower environmental temperature, and some drugs (including nicotine) lead to a higher resting metabolic rate. Basically, our only control over our metabolic rate (other than through drugs like caffeine and nicotine) is how much exercise we can squeeze into our daily routine. This is the "Energy Out" part of the equation. If you can expend as many calories as you consume, your weight will remain stable. If you consume more than you expend, you will gain weight; if you expend more than you consume, you will lose weight. It is pretty much that simple.

ENTER NICOTINE

Adding nicotine to the equation changes everything. Nicotine is a stimulant whose effects resemble those of an amphetamine, jacking up your basal metabolic rate and suppressing your appetite. It may also raise your general activity level—what one expert labeled "the fidget factor." For starters, all the rituals associated with extracting a cigarette from the pack, lighting up, and moving the cigarette back and forth between ashtray and lips undoubtedly add up to a measurable calorie expenditure over time. Then, if you have any propensity for problem eating behaviors (for example, binge eating), it is tempting to treat nicotine as an appetite-suppressing medication. As a result, as population studies have repeatedly shown, smokers weigh several pounds less than they would have weighed had they never smoked.

Now let's look at what happens to your body when you quit smoking. Weight gain has long been recognized as a distinguishing feature of nicotine withdrawal, as opposed to other drug-withdrawal syndromes. Our caloric needs rest in a very delicate balance. For most of your adult life, unless you change your smoking, eating, or exercise habits, your weight will remain relatively stable—although, as noted, it will creep up over time as your metabolism decreases with age. Stopping smoking disrupts this delicate balance. It causes a shift in your personal energy balance equation such that if you make no changes in your eating and/or activity patterns, you will probably gain weight. While the reasons for this phenomenon are not fully understood, several contributing factors have been identified:

* Very early weight gain is due, at least in part, to increases in water retention or "water weight" when the diuretic effects of nicotine are removed.

* Increased eating, especially during the early weeks of smoking abstinence, is well documented.

* As noted above, nicotine elevates resting metabolic rate, and removal of nicotine causes a reduction in resting metabolic rate.

* There may also be a decrease in general activity level— that "fidget factor" we talked about earlier—when the effects of nicotine are removed. It was recently reported that fidgeters burn up to 350 more calories per day than people who don't tap, squirm, and wriggle. Once you're past the jitters you may experience during the early stages of tobacco withdrawal, quitting may make you less of a fidgeter!

* Finally, it is clear that some women "use" nicotine to help control problem eating behaviors. Seriously disordered eating is covered in greater detail in Chapter 6.

If you took no special measures to manage your weight, how much would you gain? Population studies suggest that when people quit smoking, they gain until they reach the weight they would have weighed had they never smoked—or maybe even more, according to at least one study. The average weight gain for women has been variously reported as something on the order of 10 pounds, but it can range from zero (or even loss of weight) to well in excess of 25 or 30 pounds. How much your own weight will change depends on a variety of factors—many of which are potentially under your control.

(By the way, it should be clear now why starting smoking is not a good dieting tool. Teenagers who start smoking are unlikely to differ in weight from those who don't. We have done several studies in college women and found no difference in weight between smokers and nonsmokers in this age group. The weight-suppressing effects of smoking tend to emerge over time, by reducing normal adult weight gain so that eventually, on average, adult smokers weigh about ten pounds less than their nonsmoking counterparts. *If you are a young woman and a light smoker, and you wish to gain as little weight as possible when you quit, <u>now</u> would be a good time to stop smoking.* It is far easier to quit now than it will be later, when you're a confirmed smoker, and when you're more likely to gain weight after quitting.)

Weight gain begins almost immediately upon stopping smoking—for some women, as much as three pounds in the first week or so. After three to six months, weight gain will taper off and weight will stabilize for most women. At that point, they will fall into one of three categories:

1. Approximately a quarter will gain five pounds or less, with a handful maintaining or even losing weight.

2. Around half will gain somewhere between 5 and 15 pounds.

3. The remaining quarter will gain more than 15 pounds— with about half of these women gaining in excess of 30 pounds.

The number of pounds the mythical "average woman" will put on is far less consequential than the number of pounds *you* will put on (assuming you take no measures to counteract weight gain). Although it isn't easy to predict which of the three categories you'll end up in, the best starting estimate is

that you'll be somewhere in the 5- to 15-pound range. If you are older, if you are a heavy smoker, or if you have smoked for a long time, you may find yourself inclined to greater weight gain than younger or lighter smokers. Black women tend to gain more weight than white or Asian-American women. Perhaps surprisingly, obese women may be somewhat less susceptible to large weight gain. Some women may even be genetically programmed to gain larger amounts of weight after quitting; although additional research will be needed to confirm this finding, people with a particular form of a certain gene (the dopamine receptor gene) have been reported to show greater increases in the rewarding value of food and greater weight gain following smoking abstinence.

If you've quit for an extended period in the relatively recent past, the amount of weight you gained at that time will probably give you a good idea of what will happen when you stop smoking again—unless you make an active effort to do something different. If your mother or sister has quit smoking, her experience may also provide some clues.

Maintaining or losing weight when you stop smoking may sound like a dream scenario, and, for the lucky few, it is indeed. Unfortunately, some women experience depression in response to quitting and then suffer appetite loss in response to depression. So *losing* weight when you quit is not necessarily an unmitigated blessing—since it is a poor trade-off if you end up feeling miserable. If you have experienced episodes of depression associated with loss of appetite in the past, particularly if they followed an attempt to stop smoking, you will find information about dealing with depression in Chapter 6.

At the other end of the continuum, women who gain more than fifteen pounds may very well have been using smoking to control a tendency to overeat. If you have gained large amounts of weight during past attempts to quit smoking, or if you have ever had a tendency toward binge eating, particularly if it followed an attempt to stop smoking, you may need professional help in managing your weight. Further information about disordered eating following smoking cessation can be found in Chapter 6.

To put the nicotine story into context, remember that we already live under conditions far removed from nature's plan for keeping us at an optimal body weight. The easy availability of highly processed foods, combined with modern conveniences that reduce the need for physical activity, make it difficult for many people to control their weight—witness the current so-called epidemic of obesity in the United States and, increasingly, around the globe. Meanwhile, as we saw in Chapter 1, we're surrounded with images of impossibly skinny women and bombarded with media messages that constantly up the ante for thinness as an index of attractiveness. (If you don't believe me, rent an old Marilyn Monroe movie. She was the epitome of female beauty just a few decades ago, but to most of us now she looks, well, a little on the chunky side.) For smokers—even those without discernible eating disorders—it is all too easy to rely on nicotine to give you a little boost in countering an environment that promotes weight gain while glorifying slimness. It gives the illusion that at least you're doing *something*.

Unfortunately, that's all it is—an illusion. Using smoking to control weight is like Alice in Wonderland nibbling on one side of the mushroom, then the other, to control her size. It is just two sides of the same mushroom.

But you've made a different choice, that is, to get back into harmony with nature. To do this, as I said earlier in this chapter, you need to stop feeding the beast. I don't just mean cleansing your body of nicotine and your physiological addiction to this drug. That's part of it, of course, but you also need to shed the habits you developed and replace them with sound practices for managing your weight.

This transformation may not happen overnight, but already you're actually luckier than the lifetime nonsmoker who has fallen into a series of long-standing dysfunctional patterns. Your history as a nonsmoker is shorter, perhaps much shorter, so in some ways it should be easier for you to get it right.

For most women who want to avoid or minimize weight gain, there are three main choices:

1. You can make changes in your eating patterns.

2. You can make changes in your patterns of exercise.

3. In addition to eating less and/or exercising more, you can reframe your thinking about a modest (note that I said *modest*) weight gain.

Any one or two of these alternatives, or (ideally) all three combined, will help you become a quitter who looks great, and who feels good about herself and her body. But how much emphasis you put on each strategy is something you'll need to work out for yourself, through reflection or through trial and error. ***The best combination of strategies for <u>you</u> is the one you can sustain over the long haul.*** A three-day burst of calisthenics or fasting may begin with enthusiasm but can only end in exhaustion and discouragement. You need a lifetime plan—a dynamic plan—that you can fine-tune as you grow and your needs change.

Fortunately, even small changes, if carried out consistently, can make a big difference. Whether or not you're a smoker, even a hundred more calories per day (an extra slice of bread, for example) can add as much as ten pounds to your weight over the course of a year. The good news is that just a hundred fewer calories per day can result in losing that same ten pounds over time. Small reductions in intake (for example, not eating while preparing dinner) or increases in output (like climbing the stairs instead of taking the elevator) can be helpful in avoiding or minimizing postcessation weight gain.

How do you get from where you are to where you want to be? In the next three chapters, in order to help you reach the balance that's right for you, we'll take a closer look at each of these strategies and how you can incorporate them as painlessly and elegantly as possible into your nonsmoking lifestyle. Then, in Chapter 6 we'll identify special issues that may need to be addressed in your life to put you in the "sweet spot" and keep you there.

3

Eating Less and Enjoying It More

This book is neither a diet book nor a cookbook. Whether you follow Atkins or Weight Watchers or no diet at all, whether you're a vegetarian or an omnivore, whether you're a devotée of Carlo Petrini's Slow Food movement or Rachael Ray's speed-feed cuisine, you should be able to adapt my approach to your needs. There are no rules to follow, no "yes" lists and "no" lists—unless, of course, you wish to follow a nutritional regimen of your own choosing. Rather, the focus is on how to develop an *eating plan* that works for you and how to regain control over what you eat. It is about something many of us, sadly, have lost—a positive relationship with food.

Remember our discussion of "Energy In" and "Energy Out" in Chapter 2? If you want to prevent or minimize weight gain after you quit, the way to address the "Energy In" side of the equation is very simply: *Eat less*, or, to be more precise, take in fewer calories. **The best reduced-calorie plan for _you_ is the one you can sustain over the long haul.** Such a plan will work far better than a more stringent diet that you can't bring yourself to stick with. For a few, this may mean a complete lifestyle change. For others, it is simply a matter of substitutions or small cutbacks. You may need to experiment with different strategies in order to identify the one that's best for you.

One additional caveat: Your new way of eating, however different from or similar to your old way of eating, should be at least as nutritionally sound. While admittedly it is doubt-ful that anyone would think of switching from a moderately healthful eating regimen to, say, the "Twinkie Diet" in order to control weight gain after quitting, I feel conscience bound to add this warning!

Food is a wonderful blessing. We are designed to enjoy eating because we need it to live—to build and maintain our bodies, to fuel our activities, to allow our brains to function. Yet for many individuals, this simple pleasure has turned sour in our mouths. If you cannot remember the last time you ate with completely unalloyed pleasure, you are not alone. What a tragedy this is!

We are fortunate to live in a society where, for most, food is plentiful and easily available in more than adequate amounts. Yet this very abundance is in part our undoing. Because we evolved under conditions in which naturally occurring sug-ars were rare and seasonal, conditions in which it was to our advantage to devour as much as we could on those occasions when they were available, nature had little need to provide us with "brakes" on consumption of treats. Likewise, when our protein came from sources with legs and an aversion to being eaten, it was difficult to locate and required a considerable ex-penditure of energy to bring to the dinner table. Today, when refined sugar is as close as your nearest candy machine and meat comes in Styrofoam packages from animals bred to be fat and docile, there is no mystery why our bodies seduce us into overeating.

To make food so plentiful and ensure that few go hungry, American agriculture has transformed itself from a network of family farms into an incredibly big business that, by neces-sity, emphasizes production and storage values over taste. As a result, many Americans have a limited history of eating fresh food that is grown naturally and cooked simply. They don't know what good food is supposed to taste like. Since food preferences and prejudices are established early in life, we may sometimes find ourselves liking frozen or canned goods better than fresh foods. My own husband prefers freeze-dried coffee and instant oatmeal to the real thing.

Given that we have become a nation of overeaters trained to enjoy the taste of processed foods, is it any wonder that so many have developed an adversarial relationship with food? Or that food becomes a weapon in struggles for control between parents and children or between husbands and wives? Or that food turns into a guilty pleasure, the enemy of attractiveness, a false friend that provides comfort at the price of beauty? Or that whole classes of food are demonized because of their nutritional composition or even because of their color?

If you can relate to any of the above, the occasion of quitting smoking provides a unique opportunity to repair your relationship with food. When you start eliminating nicotine and other foul tobacco products from your body, it is a good time to think about what you are putting *into* your body.

So my first and most important dietary recommendation is to embrace a policy of *mindful eating*. Mindful eating means watching portion size, eating more slowly, chewing your food thoroughly, savoring the taste of each bite. (And remember, everything tastes and smells better when you're not smoking!) It means attention to presentation—an artful arrangement of food on the plate, harmonizing color combinations, pretty garnishes, appetizers, and soups that whet the appetite without launching an orgy of eating. It means using a smaller plate so that a normal-sized portion doesn't look so lonely. It means sitting down when you eat and adding ceremony to your meals. It means taking steps to reduce mealtime stress and consequent stress eating. Mindful eating means all of these things and more: It is an attitude, and it is a way of actively engaging with your food that expresses your unique style.

Some nutritionists will say it also means not reading at the table or having dinner in front of the television—and if you can eliminate these practices without further disrupting activities that give you satisfaction, it is probably a good idea. But if these patterns are an integral part of your little daily pleasures or your social interactions, I do not advocate creating yet another "no-no" or source of conflict for yourself or your family. Women are usually good multitaskers, and most of us can keep more than one idea in our heads at a time. (That's why we're the mothers!) In fact, it is a good practice to cultivate your ability to eat mindfully *and* do something else, whether it be to carry on a lively conversation or whatever else you may want or need to do while eating.

Amazingly, eating slowly actually helps you to eat less. This is not only for the obvious reason that eating more slowly over the same period of time results in lower food intake. It is also because eating slowly gives your digestive system and brain time to become aware that you've sent your stomach some food. If you wolf down your food, you have probably already overeaten by the time your brain gets the signal that you've met your caloric needs. Furthermore, eating mindfully and actively taking pleasure in your food will help to allay the feeling of perpetual dissatisfaction, the feeling that you haven't quite derived what you wanted or anticipated from your meal.

Here are a couple of other thoughts for you to consider:

* The need to clean your plate is deeply ingrained in some of us. In a world where millions are starving, no one wants to waste or throw out good food. But stop and reflect: Finishing everything on your plate or eating what

your children leave behind to avoid throwing it away does nothing to redress the maldistribution of food in the world and is in essence treating your body like a garbage can. Preparing and serving smaller portions, or saving even small leftovers to garnish future meals, is a better approach. If all else fails, pitching it is better than eating it when you're no longer hungry. Or as Ann, coordinator of the Nicotine Research Laboratory for many years and herself a former smoker, likes to say: "It's better as *waste* than as *waist*."

✳ We Americans have a long history of surprising foreigners with the amount of food we eat. Portion control is critical for the quitter who wants to avoid weight gain, and it may actually be easier than you think. People tend to eat what's in front of them, says Dr. Paul Rozin, a psychology professor at the University of Pennsylvania and an expert in food choices. He believes that most people could cut portion sizes by 10 percent without noticing any difference.

✳ The sad truth is that, except for exceptionally tall and large-boned women, the calorie quota required to maintain a healthy weight is rather low and discouragingly easy to meet. Women require fewer calories than men to maintain body weight, partly because of metabolic differences and partly because women are, on average, smaller than men. Be careful not to match your husband or male friend bite for bite. When he takes a second helping, it is tempting to join him—so much more sociable! Besides, it doesn't leave you longingly watching him eat. If you anticipate that this will happen, adjust your first portion accordingly or just eat much more slowly than your larger companion.

* If you slip and overeat, don't let this derail you or undermine your sense of being in charge of your eating
  behavior. Behavioral scientists call this all-too-common
  reaction the "abstinence-violation effect": "Oh, well, I've
  already eaten more than I intended; I may as well just keep
  going." One slip, or even several, won't undo all your good
  work unless you let it. Forgive yourself and move on!

* Reward yourself for doing well. Examples might include
  buying a new scarf, a good book, or flowers; watching a
  movie; or savoring a long soak in the tub. Work on iden-
  tifying nonfood and nontobacco indulgences in life that
  give particular pleasure to *you* and that you can bestow
  upon yourself to celebrate your successes.

* And though it may seem counterintuitive, food rewards
  don't have to be ruled out altogether, if you proceed with
  caution. Let's talk about that friend of so many women—
  chocolate. Dark (semisweet or bittersweet) chocolate can
  lift your mood (no surprises there), and it actually has a
  number of health benefits (really!) when taken in small
  amounts and savored. For example, one Hershey's dark
  chocolate candy kiss is twenty-five calories, one Dove
  dark chocolate piece is forty-two calories, and one square
  of Ghirardelli's dark chocolate is fifty-five calories. Ignore
  the serving sizes suggested by the manufacturers, which
  will bump you up into the two-hundred-plus calorie
  range. Think one piece, not one serving; to quote Mireille
  Guiliano, author of the best-selling book *French Women
  Don't Get Fat*, "It's all in the first bites." A restaurant near
  my home offers single-bite sundaes for dessert. What a
  cool idea! How often have you longed for "just a taste" of
  that gorgeous cheesecake or ganache and ended up with

a $7 megaserving? And more and more, single-bite serv-
ings are becoming available in packaged form as well.

* Your first line of defense is in the grocery store. Make a list
and stick to it. Don't shop when you're hungry. It is easier
to be mindful when your fridge and cupboards aren't
laden with highly caloric foods that tempt you to overeat.

* After you bring the groceries home, store calorie-dense
foods in the freezer to decrease impulse eating. (It is a
great place for your dark chocolate.)

* Holidays, times when preparing sumptuous spreads and
feasting with family and friends are an essential part of the
ritual, present a special challenge. Thanksgiving ushers
in the season that tests the resolve most severely, abetted
by the midwinter darkness. (Most people put on approximately a pound over the winter, with heavier people gaining proportionally more.) And don't forget Halloween,
a stealth holiday—one we may forget to classify as a food
trap. To get around it, don't choose your favorite goodies to
offer to trick-or-treaters. That way you won't be so tempted
to scarf up the leftovers (or to raid your stash before the
goblins even come a-knocking). Better still, do your part
to avoid passing the candy habit on to the next generation
by handing out coins or healthful treats like raisins.

* Limit your exposure to endocrine disruptors. Endocrine
disruptors are synthetic chemicals that, when absorbed
into the body, either mimic or block hormones and dis-
rupt the body's normal functions in ways that may promote obesity. Endocrine disruptors have increased in
the environment and in the food chain over the past few
decades. It would be virtually impossible to eliminate all
exposure, but here are some simple steps you can take:

* Eat organic foods.

* Avoid heating or storing food in plastic containers or plastic wrap.

* Limit the use of pesticides in your home or yard, or on your pet.

* If fish is one of your dietary staples, check with your state government to determine levels of pesticide contamination in fish from lakes, rivers, or bays and adjust your consumption accordingly.

* Restaurants—a topic in and of itself. American restaurants (sometimes, alas, in an effort to substitute quantity for quality) tend to serve humongous portions of food that encourage gorging at meals. No wonder eating frequently in restaurants doubles the risk of obesity! Good solutions include sharing a main course with your companion or making a meal of one or two appetizers. Some restaurants will allow you to order child-size portions even if your driver's license says you no longer qualify. Eat a low-calorie snack before leaving home, then ask your waiter to hold the bread and bring you a glass of sparkling water instead while waiting for your meal. The "doggie bag" solution works much better, I've found, if you ask your waiter to bag the other half of your meal *before* rather than after serving it on your plate. (Someone who read this book in manuscript form was incredulous and asked me if I'd ever really done that. The answer is, "Yes, many times," and the request has always been graciously received.) If the restaurant is an upscale one that prides itself on presentation, a better approach is to ask the waiter to bring you the take-out container along with your food—and then pack up your "leftovers" before beginning your meal.

A word about food and mood. Although you'll sometimes see bloggers describing their current mood as "hungry," hunger *per se* is not a mood. It can, however, affect your mood. My cats, Tabasco and Marshmallow, are accustomed to being fed at 5:00 PM. Sometime around 4:00 or 4:30, they become extremely active. Although most of the time they're the greatest of buddies, around mealtime they often wrestle and roughhouse and occasionally even hiss at each other. If I'm working, they leap up on my desk and push knickknacks onto my keyboard. Once they've had their dinner, they settle down and eventually become quite somnolent. If my husband and I watch a DVD in the evening, they curl up between us on the sofa and purr. The same cycle of premeal activation used to play itself out in our bedroom before the morning feeding— until my husband tired of the feline alarm clock and banished them to the basement overnight.

Similarly, parents of young children often notice that crankiness and whining increase in proportion to the time since the last meal, and that a well-timed snack can usually defuse the situation. Adults, too—some more than others—can become crabby and irritable when they're hungry. Does this remind you of cigarette cravings? It is no coincidence. Nicotine commandeers many of the biological mechanisms designed to tell you to *do something about it* when you're hungry. If you're someone who experiences serious "food swings," prepare to stave off hunger attacks by carrying low-calorie munchies in your purse or briefcase, or eat five or six small meals per day rather than three. Don't wait till you start snapping at your spouse or coworkers, which can only make matters worse (and even tempt you to seek solace in food).

THE EATING-SMOKING CONNECTION

So far we've talked mostly about weight-management strategies that apply to anyone, regardless of smoking status. Now let's focus on some particular trouble spots you may face as a former or soon-to-be former smoker.

When smokers are asked which cigarette of the day would be most difficult one for them to give up, by far the two most common responses are "the first cigarette of the day" or "the one I smoke at the end of a meal." "With coffee" and "with alcohol" are also right up there among the top choices.

An excellent alternative to smoking upon awakening is none other than to eat a good breakfast. Skipping breakfast may intuitively feel like an easy way to avoid consuming the most boring calories of the day and save room for more tempting goodies later on, but it is not a sound weight-management strategy and, in fact, is often self-defeating: Eating at regular intervals, when your body expects food, helps prevent the appetite surge that many women experience later in the day. Shop specifically for "what sounds good" or for what is convenient first thing in the morning. Prepare as much of your breakfast as you can the night before to minimize the delay between waking and eating. Get your coffeemaker going as soon as possible, or put it on a timer you can set the night before. Give your breakfast as much eye, nose, and taste appeal as you can. Entice yourself with whatever it takes until you've established the breakfast habit; you can aim for variety later, after you've tired of your routine. If you have a partner or child who is very supportive of your effort to stop smoking without gaining weight, he or she may be willing to pamper you by bringing you breakfast in bed that first week, complete with folded cloth napkin. ("Dream on," I can hear some of you saying!)

Unfortunately, food and tobacco often go hand in hand. (In fact, with the introduction and enforcement of clean indoor air policies, a few chichi New York restaurants experimented—mercifully briefly—with tobacco as a dessert ingredient to satisfy their smoking customers' desire to end the meal with a dose of nicotine.) The after-dinner cigarette has probably become somewhat less compelling in an era when many private homes as well as public places have gone "smoke-free"; still, it is a time when many women miss their smoke or, alternatively, may be tempted to substitute a calorie-laden dessert. One solution is to get up from the table and do something else. (Flossing or brushing your teeth, for example, gives you something to do with your hands and will please your dentist as well.)

Leaping up from the dinner table to floss your teeth, however, may not strike you as being exactly in the spirit of mindful eating. An alternative is to find some other low- or noncaloric way to signal to your body that the meal is over and to effect a smooth transition from dinner to *après*-dinner. If you don't already take tea or coffee at the end of your evening meal, for example, now might be a good time to start doing so—preferably without a lot of sugar and cream, and preferably decaf. Make a small ritual of the brewing process. Or adopt the French way of ending a meal: Serve your salad *after* the main course—followed, *mais oui*, by a small portion of fruit. (The French are world champions when it comes to mindful eating and also when it comes to staying slim, so they should know! Even at fast-food restaurants, they spend more time at the table than Americans do. Unfortunately, they are also pretty good at smoking, or at least they have been up until recently—a puzzling fact but one far less worthy of imitation.)

Ending the meal with a sweet is less desirable because refined sugar can lead to an insulin overshoot that stimulates a desire for *more* sugar. If you are a confirmed dessert eater and don't find a meal complete without one, however, identify low-calorie treats like a meringue or a frozen fudge bar, a piece of fruit, or desserts made with a sugar substitute. As a general rule, cutting down on your intake of refined sugar is helpful in controlling appetite as well as weight.

The same general logic applies to cigarettes smoked along with coffee and alcohol. Just as you eat mindfully, you can also *drink* mindfully. Remember that alcohol breaks down inhibitions of all kinds, including your resolve to avoid smoking and reduce food intake. It is also a source of empty calories, so going for quality rather than quantity in your alcohol consumption may be a good approach for those who drink regularly. Indeed, you may find that absent the stimulant effects of nicotine, the sedating effects of alcohol are enhanced—another good reason for cutting back.

A particularly thorny problem is that you are trying to reduce caloric intake at a time when you're experiencing increased appetite. This is a perfect example of life not being fair! Even if you're determined not to gain a single pound, you may find some of the information in Chapter 5, on ways to prevent early weight gain, helpful in getting you over the hump, the peak period of increased appetite. Finally, develop a repertoire of low-calorie treats that you enjoy and can substitute for either smoking or for eating more highly caloric snacks.

WHEN TO START WORKING ON YOUR EATING PATTERNS

More research is needed to establish the best time to begin trying to control your weight when you're trying to stop smoking. Meanwhile, you need to make a decision about how to proceed. Fortunately, you don't need to know what is optimal for most people, only for yourself—and a little bit of introspection may help you decide which of the following approaches is likely to work best for you:

Option 1: Put your weight concerns on hold until you've successfully stopped smoking and then (when you know just how bad things really are—or, maybe, when you discover that they are not as bad as your worst fears) attack the problem of weight management. The sequential approach has often been advocated by behavior therapists, whose mantra has been "work on one problem at a time." This approach has good scientific support and may work best for many smokers. If you can face the prospect of deferring dietary changes until you are past the worst of the withdrawal effects of smoking cessation—*even if it means tolerating some initial weight gain*—then the "wait-and-see" approach may be the right one for you. Women who are invested in staying slim, however—a group that probably includes most readers of this book—may find this approach distressing and likely to undermine rather than reinforce their attempt to stop smoking.

Option 2: Making your target quit date for smoking also your target date for modifying your eating habits may appeal to you if you like the challenge of addressing two problem behaviors at once (some people do) and see tackling them both at the same time as part of a more general "cleansing" operation. Be aware that there is little evidence to support the proposition that combining weight control and smoking cessation increases the likelihood of succeeding at either. On the other hand, although caloric restriction increases nicotine intake in smokers not trying to quit, addressing weight concerns at the start of a quit attempt does not appear to impede quitting. If you are convinced it is the right way for you—as I suspect will be the case for many readers of this book—then I see no reason not to trust your instincts.

Option 3: An approach that many weight-concerned women smokers come up with on their own is to diet off pounds *before* you quit ("a cushion for the expected weight gain," as one woman put it). If you do this with the idea that you can then resume your normal eating patterns and end up weighing what you did before you quit, this strategy may get you past the difficult initial days of abstinence from smoking, but in the long run you are probably doomed to disappointment. Moreover, there is a danger that you will internalize and become "bonded" to your new, lower body weight and still resist quitting. I strongly advise against crash dieting as a prelude to a quit attempt. If you see your new way of eating as a lifetime commitment, however, then by all means start working on the mindful eating approach before you quit. In fact, taking charge of your eating style will probably make it easier to control the increased urge to eat right after you quit and increase your confidence about quitting smoking as well. Peg your quit attempt, however, not to a set amount of weight loss but rather to your feeling of confidence in your new eating style.

In the next chapter, I'll address "Energy Out" and ways of increasing your physical activity without turning yourself into an Olympic athlete. Like controlling "Energy In," it requires a thoughtful and respectful approach. But also like controlling "Energy In," it is not impossibly difficult or beyond the reach of most women. Mastering these techniques will increase your self-respect and make you feel good about yourself.

Exercise—Minimizing Gain with Minimal Pain

Fitness training, working out, aerobics—whatever term its proponents concoct to give it a little more cachet, exercise by any other name is still exercise. For many of us, it is a word that brings groans to the lips and strikes guilt in the soul.

If you want to prevent or minimize post-cessation weight gain, the way to address the Energy Out side of the equation is very simply: *Exercise more*—or to be more precise, expend more calories. ***The best increased-activity plan for you is the one you can sustain over the long haul.*** Sound familiar? It should, because the same principles I suggested for decreasing food intake apply to increasing physical activity.

Unlike eating, however, nature did not have to make physical activity feel good in order to persuade us to do it. To obtain food and escape from harm under precivilized conditions required us to move our bodies. The connection of activity with survival was immediate and obvious, and those who failed to do so didn't live very long. Although exercise actually does enhance mood, the effect is sufficiently subtle that we may fail to recognize or cultivate it unless we train ourselves to do so. In short, most of us are not particularly motivated to move our bodies unnecessarily and are easily deterred from doing so. ("I should exercise, but it's too hot." "I should exercise, but who has time?" You know the drill.)

Just as modern civilization tends to discourage dietary restraint, so too it discourages exercise. We have become very clever at inventing labor-saving devices and modes of transportation that "save" our personal energy. We've traded in our washboards for washing machines and buy our butter in handy packages instead of churning it from cream as our great-great-grandmothers once did. In school, if you belong to an older generation, "phys ed" probably consisted of team sports that are difficult to carry into adulthood because they require specialized equipment or coordinating with other people's schedules, or because prolonged engagement in them results in wear and tear on the joints that eventually leads to discontinuation. If you belong to a younger generation, "phys ed" may have been optional or nonexistent. All this may be changing as our collective consciousness has been raised about our national epidemic of obesity, but it is too late to help those who are now adults.

It is not too late, however, to find your way to a physical activity plan that works for you—maybe even something you look forward to. For some women, this is not a problem, but I can hear others muttering, "Impossible!" I might have said so myself at one time. I grew up in a sedentary household; my father's idea of a fun family outing was going to the local airport on Sunday afternoons to watch people flying model airplanes. But watching my mother die of a stroke at the age of fifty-two frightened me, and watching my husband taking obvious pleasure in physical activity inspired me. Between the carrot and the stick, I have managed to develop and maintain for decades an exercise routine that I not only tolerate but actually enjoy. For over twenty years I ran daily, sometimes with a friend, sometimes with my husband, sometimes with a headset tuned to NPR. Often our dog came along. Eventually I switched to step aerobics, which I now do three or four times per week, interspersed with exercise videos, a recumbent bike in my basement, and a weekly walking date with a group of women friends. If I can do it, trust me, so can you.

Up to 70 percent of beginning exercisers fall by the wayside within nine months. Be honest and realistic if you want to end up in the remaining 30 percent. Start by thinking carefully about your exercise preferences. Do you like to work out alone, with one or two like-minded others, or with a group? Do you enjoy competitive sports or less structured activities? Do you prefer rhythmic activity accompanied by music, listening to the radio as you work out, or just communing with yourself in silence? Would you rather work out in the morning or the afternoon, or in three or four mini-sessions spread out across the day? Does the thought of working out in front of a mirror make your heart sink, or do you like the feedback you get from watching your body move? Do you have any physical limitations that dictate the activities you can and cannot do?

Once you have narrowed down your preferences, think about your options for carrying them out. Is there a gym that's accessible to you? Do you have room in your home to exercise? If, like me, you're a fan of exercise videos and DVDs, do you have a television and videocassette or DVD player available where you wish to work out? If your preferred exercise requires lots of specialized equipment, or if it requires being outdoors, do you have alternatives for times when the gym is closed or the weather is inclement or your walking partner is on vacation? (Check out your local shopping malls; some of them open early for walkers.) Can you make or share baby-sitting arrangements, or does your gym have child care available? Try to anticipate and think your way around any barriers that you might be tempted to use as excuses not to exercise "just this once." Enrolling in and paying for a class—Pilates, Jazzercise, step aerobics—can help provide an additional incentive to attend regularly. Look over my list of "Additional Reading and Resources for Weight and Mood Management" at the end of this book to help identify options that map onto your preferences. Especially if you've never exercised before, have an injury or infirmity that precludes weight-bearing exercise, are tight on space for working out, or simply dislike the sensation of moving your body around the room, be sure to check out Jodi Stolove's amazing *Chair Dancing* video/DVD series. In my opinion, this series offers the ideal starter exercise program for any "adult-onset exerciser" who is no longer young and agile.

As you design your exercise routine, try to include the following types of exercise (not necessarily all on the same day!), both for variety and to allow your body time to recover:

* *Aerobic exercise* is any large-muscle activity that you can sustain for two to three minutes or longer, forcing your heart and lungs to work in order to obtain oxygen from the air. Examples of aerobic activities are walking, dancing, gardening, raking or mowing the lawn, hiking, bicycling, lap swimming, jogging, distance running (look for that "endorphin high!"), tennis, basketball, and cross-country skiing. These activities can increase your metabolic rate by a factor of five to twenty times the energy you expend sitting down.

* *Resistance exercise,* also known as strength training, contributes to nicely toned muscles and boosts metabolism. Some women fear that weight lifting will make them look like bodybuilders. Not to worry: Sharply chiseled, bulging muscles are difficult for men to achieve and even more

so for women; this will never happen without extraordinary and focused effort on your part. Methods for resistance training include free weights, weight machines, and calisthenics (e.g., push-ups, sit-ups, chin-ups). In isotonic exercise—for example, lifting weights—a body part is moved, and the muscle shortens or lengthens. Isometric exercise, by contrast, is a type of strength training involving contracting your muscles without moving—for example, pressing your palms against a wall. Strength training is often done in sets of eight repetitions or "reps." A complete workout typically lasts around thirty minutes and involves a series of exercises using different muscle groups.

* *Flexibility exercise* involves gentle stretching to increase the length of your muscles and range of motion in your joints. It may consist of a series of specific stretching exercises or be part of a yoga, dance, or aerobics class. Because one of the main goals of stretching is to lengthen the connective tissue surrounding your muscle fibers, flexibility exercises should be done after you've already warmed up your muscles with a few minutes of aerobic activity. A typical session involves a minute or two on each stretching exercise. Regular stretching helps to maintain your mobility and can also improve your posture.

As with eating, an important strategy in developing an exercise routine you can live with is to exercise *mindfully*. Pay attention to your body as you work out. Tune into the way your mood lifts as you continue your activity. Make sure you wear clothes that are comfortable to move in and make you feel good about your body. Reward yourself with a satisfying stretch during or at the end of your workout.

As noted above, exercise at any time of day is better than no exercise. Although experts argue among themselves about the relative merits of morning versus evening exercise, morning exercise works best for me, and I have lots of company: People who exercise consistently tend to be morning exercisers. Exercising in the morning ensures that your workout won't get crowded out by other demands if the day becomes hectic. If you're not a "morning person," a morning workout may appeal because it is over before you're fully awake! But if exercise at noontime or after work is a better fit for your schedule or your desires, go for it—or change the timing each day.

"But what about other forms of physical activity?" you may be wondering. It is hard for most of us to get enough exercise via our daily activities on a regular basis, but strenuous fat-burning activities such as gardening or mowing the lawn (if you use the kind of mower you push around), for example, certainly count toward your exercise quota.

It is also wise to think about ways to reduce sitting as well. Surprised? Says Dr. Frank Hu, professor of nutrition and epidemiology at the Harvard School of Public Health, "For most people, it is not sufficient to address only the exercise side of the coin. Equally important is the sedentary side of the coin." So get up and walk around. Instead of e-mailing, walk to your coworker's office. Go to your child's room rather than yelling up the stairs. Wear shoes that will allow you to take advantage of opportunities to do a little extra walking. Wear a pedometer to help motivate walking. Park at the far end of the lot. Take the stairs rather than the elevator. (Stair climbing can burn a whopping 1,100 calories/hour!) One of my favorite cartoons shows a group of people in sweat suits waiting for an elevator to take them to the gym—ignoring the immediately adjacent staircase!

THE EXERCISE-SMOKING CONNECTION

Now that we've reviewed some general strategies for developing an exercise routine you can live with, let's talk about some ways that you can use exercise to help you become and remain a nonsmoker without gaining weight.

In Chapter 2 we discussed the difficulty of giving up that first cigarette of the day, and I recommended making a beeline for the breakfast table. Another option is to start your day by exercising. Not only does grabbing your running shoes provide an alternative to grabbing a cigarette, but exercise can also substitute for a cigarette in "getting things moving."

While very strenuous exercise suppresses appetite in men, it may actually backfire for women and lead to increased compensatory eating—a situation further complicated by the effects of stopping smoking. If you find you are ravenous when you finish your workout, experiment with modulating your activity level until you find an intensity and duration of exercise that reduces rather than increases your appetite. Another important recommendation: Never go thirsty when you exercise; keep plenty of drinking water on hand. If you're hungry or anticipate a strenuous workout, have a small snack before starting. Snacks that combine carbohydrates with protein and are small enough to eat prior to exercising include peanut butter with apple slices, tortilla chips and bean dip, hummus on veggies, or yogurt with cereal.

In addition to its other virtues, exercise can help you combat cravings for a cigarette and smoking withdrawal symptoms such as depression, anxiety, restlessness, and inability to concentrate. Exercise, like smoking, releases stimulatory substances called catecholamines in your body. Obviously you won't always be in a position to jump up and do calisthenics when the urge to smoke strikes. Fortunately, a few minutes of isometrics are often enough to get you over the "hump." If you can, keep a small set of hand weights or a Dyna-Band (a resistant elastic exercise band) handy for a five-minute mini-workout. If all else fails, do your Kegels (that is, tightening and relaxing the muscles of the pelvic floor; you can isolate these muscles by starting and stopping the flow when urinating).

WHEN TO START INCREASING YOUR PHYSICAL ACTIVITY

Like mindful eating, incorporating a program of mindful exercise into your lifestyle is something that can be done as soon as you're ready. If you can establish a regular routine of physical activity before you quit smoking, it will be helpful in enhancing your mood, building your confidence, and dealing with withdrawal symptoms.

Especially if you're not used to physical activity, it is a good idea to build up gradually, over the course of a few weeks. Once you actually stop smoking, your exercise routine will become easier and more pleasurable as your lungs clear and your aerobic capacity increases.

As I have already said (but it bears repeating), getting your body into gear—and liking it!—requires a thoughtful and respectful approach. It is a challenge, certainly, but it is a challenge that many people have met successfully. Controlling your food intake makes you feel empowered; getting the exercise you need makes you feel empowered *and*, once acclimated, makes you feel good while you're doing it.

SO HOW MUCH EXERCISE DO I NEED?

To maintain your precessation weight, you need to increase your caloric expenditure by eating less, exercising more, or both. (If you're overweight or obese, you may be hoping not just to maintain but to lose weight. This situation will be dealt with in greater detail in Chapter 6.) So the question here is not about how much exercise you should be doing but about how much *more* exercise you should be doing to bridge the gap between your smoking and postcessation caloric needs. The answer to this question lies in some combination of how much less you are eating and how heavy a smoker you were. Unfortunately, the world is still waiting for a formula for computing the calorie deficit required for postcessation weight maintenance in a given individual. Meanwhile, the most important principle is: Choose the form of exercise you *will* do (and *keep on* doing). A goal that you can't sustain is worse than no goal at all.

When you think about increasing your exercise level, take these three components into account: duration, frequency, and intensity. A few years ago, the government issued guidelines recommending at least half an hour of vigorous exercise per day for fitness and sixty to ninety minutes per day for weight management. This advice rightly provoked considerable controversy. In fact, the amount of exercise needed for weight management varies widely from person to person and for some people may actually be less than they need to achieve aerobic fitness. The amount of exercise needed to enhance mood is even less. You would never have known this from the guidelines, however, which seemed calculated to defeat most people before they even got out of their chairs

In 2008 new guidelines were issued, and, fortunately, this time sanity prevailed. Adults aged eighteen to sixty-four are now advised to do a minimum of two hours and thirty minutes per week of moderately intense exercise, seventy-five minutes of vigorous aerobic activity, or some combination of the two, with additional health benefits accruing if you can do more.

Importantly, unlike the rigid formula specifying a long daily bout of activity, much more discretion is now allowed in distributing activity throughout the week, provided individual episodes last at least ten minutes. Engaging in moderate or high-intensity muscle-strengthening activities that involve all major muscle groups on two or more days per week is also advised.

If you're out of shape or out of practice, even the amount of exercise recommended by the newest version of the guidelines may seem daunting. Again, choose the type and amount of exercise you *will* do (and *keep on* doing), not the exercise the government (or anyone else) thinks you should do. Once you've established an exercise pattern you enjoy, and your lung function is no longer compromised by smoking, you may find yourself motivated to inch closer toward goals specified in the guidelines. But remember: You want to increase your exercise level enough to maintain your precessation weight, not qualify for the Olympics.

Exercise of "moderate intensity" is generally what is recommended, and moderation sounds good, right? But what the heck is moderate? Well, the American College of Sports Medicine helpfully provides two useful ways out of this dilemma. One requires no equipment at all; the other requires only a watch or clock and a modest facility for mental arithmetic. Either method will provide adequate reassurance that your workout is giving you enough of, well, a workout.

The first and easiest method is the "Rate of Perceived Exertion" (RPE), sometimes called the Borg scale. RPE is a subjective rating system that's about as low-tech as it gets. The original system used a scale ranging from 6 to 19 to measure the intensity of a workout, as follows: 6–8 very, very light; 9–10 very light; 11–12 fairly light; 13–14 somewhat hard; 15–16 hard;

17–18 very hard; 19 very, very hard. Aerobics instructors often modify this to a more intuitively satisfying scale ranging from 1 to 10, with 6–7 being the target zone for moderate-intensity exercise. The idea is to hone in on the physical sensations you experience when you exercise, including increases in heart rate, breathing rate, sweating, and muscle fatigue, and translate the result into an estimate of how hard you're working. This system may strike you as a little illogical—"I think it's moderate exercise, so it must be moderate exercise"—but it does have the advantage of encouraging you to focus on how exercise affects the way you feel and actually correlates fairly well with other measures of exertion, especially in experienced users.

The second method is based on the percentage of your maximum heart rate that you reach during your workout. To use this method, you'll have to learn to find your pulse either in your wrist or in your carotid artery, which is located on the side of your neck. You also need a watch that measures seconds and a calculator (just the first time). Use the watch to see how many heartbeats you count in six seconds at a high point in your workout. Multiply that number by ten to obtain your heart rate in beats per minute. After that, calculate your maximum heart rate. Assuming you're not taking drugs that lower your heart rate (as do many blood pressure medications), an approximation can be computed by subtracting your age from 220. If your heart rate (beats per minute) at the peak of your workout falls somewhere between 55 percent and 69 percent of that number, you're probably in the sweet spot. Here is an example that puts all of this together: If your age is 35, your maximum heart rate would be $220 - 35 = 185$. Fifty-five percent of 185 is 102, and 69 percent is 128, so your target range would be 102–128 beats per minute, or somewhere between 10 and 13 beats for a six-second reading.

One question that sometimes arises: How accurate are the LED calorie-counter displays on exercise equipment? The answer: Not very. The timers are generally accurate, and there is no reason why the number of revolutions shouldn't be. But even if you plug in your weight, height, and age, the calorie counters are imprecise at best. To convince yourself of this, try two or three machines of different brands, and I predict they'll vary considerably in how optimistic an estimate of calorie expenditure they provide. If you use the same machine every day, however, you can probably be confident that if the machine tells that you expended more calories today than yesterday, you probably did. And since *more* is your goal, the readout can be useful as a relative measure.

WHAT IF YOU'RE ALREADY MAXED OUT ON EXERCISE?

Most of this chapter applies to that majority of women who don't exercise enough and find it hard to work up much enthusiasm about increasing their activity level. But what about women who already exercise a lot? Raphaela, one of the project coordinators at the Nicotine Research Laboratory, for example, is a semiprofessional ballerina, and a number of her dancer colleagues smoke to help control their weight. They have regular weigh-ins, and their jobs are threatened if they put on a few pounds. This is a job requirement, not just for cosmetic reasons, but because male dancers need to be able to hoist them. Other professions or avocations that pressure women to be thin include modeling, gymnastics, ice skating, and horseback riding. These are very specific and sometimes extreme situations, but even readers whose jobs don't demand thinness may already have gotten the message about exercise and feel they are already doing as much as they really can.

A good starting place might be to conduct an inventory of your current physical activity. Are you really doing as much as you think? To return to the smoking ballerinas: Ballet actually consists of very short bursts of energy—maximum four minutes. An average ballet class burns two hundred to four hundred calories—an okay but not great workout. To take another example, yoga may be terrific for body and soul, but, although it contributes somewhat to your overall caloric expenditure, most types of yoga aren't the best way to burn calories. So if yoga is your main fitness routine, you may need to think about supplementing it with other, more-aerobic activities, adopting modifications aimed at increasing fat-burning, or doing your Warrior and Downward-Facing Dog Poses between sets.

The next step is to determine whether, with little or no additional investment of time, you could modify your routine to punch up the intensity of your workout. How about lifting hand weights while riding an exercycle or quickening your walking pace? Or doing some crunches during commercials? Or stretching your family time by finding a group activity in which everyone can participate? Look for small changes you can make in your daily routine to expend a few more calories: taking the stairs instead of the elevator or parking a little farther from your destination. One of my colleagues takes her cell phone and walks briskly around the neighborhood while participating in conference calls—talk about multitasking!

Finally, consider using some of the money you're saving by not smoking ($1,825 per year for a pack-a-day smoker, if you pay $5 a pack) to buy a session or two with a personal trainer. A trainer can help you find ways to make the most efficient use of your exercise time. (You can learn more about choosing a personal trainer in the "Additional Reading and Resources for Weight and Mood Management" section at the end of this book.) This is a great way to invest positively in yourself.

Once you quit smoking, you will happily discover that you have increased lung capacity and enhanced physical performance—which may actually make it easier to "go that extra mile." If continuing the activities you're doing and doing them even better is an important goal, then quitting smoking will help you achieve it.

5

Gaining a Little and Getting Okay with It

If fear of gaining weight when you stop smoking makes you reluctant to consider quitting, you probably already know you have lots of company.

Something my colleagues and I at the Nicotine Research Laboratory started doing early on was simply asking this question of *all* the volunteers we screened for *any* study, "How much weight would you be willing to gain if you quit smoking?" These were not necessarily people who were trying to quit; they were just members of the general smoking public. The majority of the men we asked were willing to gain ten or twenty pounds. By contrast, 75 percent of the women said they were unwilling to gain more than five pounds; the most common single response, given by 40 percent of the women, was zero. Although women under twenty-five, overweight women, and severe dieters were predictably the most resistant to the prospect of weight gain, we found that, even among women *not* in these categories, there were still substantial numbers who were simply unwilling to gain more than five pounds. A smoking cessation clinic participant quoted by Klesges and DeBon in *How Women Can Finally Stop Smoking* (Hunter House, 1994) summed it up nicely: "Three pounds, and I'm outta here!"

Shortly after we published our study on willingness to tolerate postcessation weight gain, I presented our findings to a group of journalists. One reporter was so interested that he went back and did a phone survey in a much larger sample of women smokers. His results were remarkably similar to mine, which probably makes me one of the few researchers whose findings have been replicated by the *Washington Post*!

When you ask smokers directly whether they "use" smoking to control their weight, similar results emerge: Up to 40 percent of women endorse weight control as an important motive for smoking—again, compared with only a handful of the men.

For all of these reasons, I have long been skeptical of the "attitude adjustment" approach to persuading weight-concerned women to stop smoking, which generally includes telling them they'd have to gain thirty, fifty, or even a hundred pounds to equal the health hazards of smoking. Despite the documented reluctance of many women to gain even a small number of pounds, the fundamental, deep-down problem is uncertainty about whether weight gain can easily be contained, and dread that the process will spin out of control. Hearing about the thirty or fifty pounds you would have to gain (read: *might gain* or even *will probably gain*) and the image it evokes of "that future shadow"—reminiscent of the old Lucky Strike ads we talked about earlier—is hardly reassuring!

Remember that the *average* weight gain is around ten pounds. *Average* does not mean that every quitter gains ten pounds. As you learned in your grade-school arithmetic class, the average is calculated by adding together the weight gained by each quitter, ranging from zero to many times ten pounds, and then dividing that number by the total number of quitters. Metabolic changes account for a few of those pounds; the rest have to do with behavioral factors that you can control. *The trick is to keep your weight gain on the low side of the average.*

Every woman has to identify her own comfort zone, but if you're not sure where to draw the line, let me make the following suggestion: Keep your weight gain to within one unit of your body mass index, or BMI, a widely used measure of weight corrected for height. BMI is discussed in much greater detail in Chapter 6, under the topic of obesity, so read ahead if you prefer to make a precise calculation. For present purposes, however, suffice it to say that for most women, a BMI unit is in the range of five to seven pounds—closer to five if you're short, closer to seven if you're taller. It is less than a dress size (usually estimated to be around eight pounds worth), so you shouldn't need to buy a whole new wardrobe—unless, of course, you want to!

As we saw in Chapter 2, weight gain begins almost immediately upon stopping smoking, a fact that fuels the fear of runaway weight gain. The majority of attempts to quit fail within the first few days after quitting, and although the other withdrawal effects and the craving for cigarettes undoubtedly contribute to early relapse, watching the needle on the scale creep upward also takes its toll, especially among women. (Remember "Three pounds, and I'm outta here"?)

So right up front is a good time to bolster your confidence that you can maintain control over the process. Here are some steps you can take:

* If you are a menstruating woman, set your "target quit date"—the first day of your quit attempt—to occur right after the last day of your period. That way, the fluid retention associated with the critical first few days of abstinence isn't compounded by the bloating and weight gain that often occur just before and during the menstrual

period. And, regardless of the cycle phase in which you quit, be attuned to your menstrual cycle and "inoculate" yourself psychologically against surrendering to the mood swings that may occur at this time.

* To replace the diuretic effects of nicotine, emphasize fruits, vegetables, and low-fat dairy products in the first few days after quitting—a diet that promotes the elimination of salt from the body and increases urine production.

* Try to get enough sleep. Believe it or not, getting too little sleep makes it harder to control weight. Sleep loss affects secretion of several hormones involved in appetite regulation and increases fat storage by interfering with your body's ability to metabolize carbohydrates. (I swear I can detect a decrease in overnight weight loss when I've had inadequate sleep!) Tired people are hungry people, and we all know what hungry people do. Besides, you can't eat and you can't smoke while you're sleeping! To improve sleep, experts advise not eating a large meal just before bedtime, not exercising just before bedtime, avoiding caffeine (coffee, tea, and many soft drinks) late in the day, and not napping during the day. Purposefully arranging your schedule to allow for a little extra pillow time for the first week after you quit can enhance your feeling of empowerment. Try to avoid unplanned oversleeping, however. Finding yourself in an unexpected time crunch will just leave you feeling stressed and can undermine your resolve.

* Keep the indoor temperature as cool in the winter and as warm in the summer as you can comfortably tolerate. Not only is this good for the planet and for your heating/cooling bills, it can also contribute to energy expenditure that doesn't require eating less and exercising more—because

it takes you out of the "thermo-neutral zone" in which your body doesn't have to expend any energy to keep you warm or cold. It also suppresses appetite.

* Keep low-calorie munchies on hand for snack attacks or for when you feel a strong urge to put *something* in your mouth. Or try "puffing" on a cinnamon stick!

* Limit your alcohol intake. Better still, avoid it altogether for those first few days. Alcohol tends to undermine control and release your inhibitions—for eating as well as for smoking. It is also a source of empty calories. Avoid parties and bars where you'll be tempted to drink—and to smoke.

What about caffeine? Although new quitters are sometimes advised to limit caffeine intake, the basis for this recommendation is not clear. Regarding its impact on weight and appetite, claims and counterclaims lead to the conclusion that the effects, if any, are subtle. Caffeine in moderation does not appear to be particularly harmful, so if you enjoy your cuppa joe, there is no need to deprive yourself of that pleasure. A few caveats are in order, however: First, when you stop smoking, caffeine is metabolized more slowly, so you may find you need less to get the same effect. Second, sugar and cream can add up to a noticeable proportion of your daily caloric intake. Third, because smoking and coffee drinking often go hand in hand, coffee may serve as a signal to light up. Bottom line: Drink your coffee mindfully. Stay attuned to its effects on your body and the possible need to adjust your intake. Consider changing when and where you drink coffee to break down the associations between smoking and caffeine intake.

A brief note about scales: Although other forms of self-monitoring (recording food intake, measuring the intensity of exercise, etc.) are generally encouraged in behavior change programs, for some reason daily weighing has gotten a bum rap. People in weight management programs are often told, on the basis of virtually no scientific evidence, that daily weighing promotes excessive concentration on the numbers and that there is too much variability or "bounce" to give an accurate picture of weight trends. They are instructed to weigh themselves weekly, if at all. A recent study, however, suggests that this potentially useful tool may have been unjustly maligned. Among both dieters and people seeking to prevent weight gain, people who frequently weighed themselves did better than those who did not. Although this does not prove that self-weighing produced the superior results—it may simply be that the more highly motivated individuals were more prone to self-weighing—it certainly suggests that if you are among the many women for whom stepping on the bathroom scale each morning is as routine as brushing your teeth, there is no reason why you should stop doing so. Just try to weigh yourself at the same time each day, and in the same state of dress or undress.

Nicotine replacement products and Zyban all help to diminish weight gain. Zyban (which is also marketed as Wellbutrin, an antidepressant) requires a doctor's prescription, as do nicotine nasal spray and the nicotine inhaler, but nicotine gum, patches, and lozenges are available over the counter. You might consider using nicotine gum instead of the generally preferred patch, since the gum may have a greater impact on postcessation weight gain than the patch (and since having gum in your mouth is incompatible with eating!). Nicotine replacement products and Zyban have been successfully used in combination. (Note, however, that Zyban is contraindicated in people with a history of eating disorders because it may increase the possibility of seizures in such individuals.)

Unfortunately, once you stop using these products, you will lose their weight-suppressing effects. But using them from the start and then continuing to use them for several weeks as recommended by the manufacturer will confer the following benefits:

1. Their weight-suppressing effects will give you the psychological boost you need during the first few days to let you know that you're in charge of your body and not the other way around.

2. By the time you're ready to wean yourself, you'll be well established as a nonsmoker and ready to address weight issues without the additional distraction of an intense desire to smoke and discomfort from other withdrawal symptoms.

Do you have to discontinue use of these products? Good question. After all, no one expects to stop taking medications for chronic conditions like diabetes or high blood pressure after a few weeks and have the effects persist. Most smoking cessation medications, however, have been tested and marketed for short-term use. Longer-term use remains controversial, and there is no certainty that their weight-suppressing effects would be sustained indefinitely. (The antidepressant Prozac, for example, initially reduces appetite and weight in many individuals but tends to lose its weight-suppressing effects after several months of use.)

What about Chantix, the "next big thing" in smoking cessation treatment? A recent review found no evidence that Chantix reduced postcessation weight gain at end of treatment, though one study in which successful quitters received twelve additional weeks of treatment showed a modest suppression of weight. Even if Chantix does not appear to suppress postcessation weight gain, as most of the evidence suggests, it may still be a good choice for some people precisely because it is less likely to result in *delayed* weight gain when they stop taking it. Moreover, its effectiveness in suppressing craving for a cigarette may allow you to deal more effectively with other withdrawal symptoms, such as increased appetite. The possibility of combining Chantix with a nicotine replacement product, which could add a weight-suppressing component to Chantix treatment, has so far been tested only in an inpatient setting, and, as of this writing, the manufacturer advises against doing so.

Concerns about possible serious psychiatric side effects of both Zyban and Chantix have recently prompted the FDA to require warning labels on the packaging of these products. A more extended discussion of pharmacotherapy for smoking, including safety issues and other factors that may affect your choice of medication, appears in Chapter 7, "Quitting for Good," along with a chart giving clinical information about all Food and Drug Administration (FDA)–approved medications.

A note of caution: If, despite your best efforts, you find yourself gaining more weight or gaining weight faster than you had anticipated, or if you cannot control your eating, *please* don't try to solve the problem by returning to smoking. Skip ahead to the sections dealing with large weight gain and disordered eating in Chapter 6. Check out the "Additional Reading and Resources for Weight and Mood Management" section at the end of this book. Get professional help if necessary.

Finally, taking the longer view: Remember that regardless of smoking status, most Americans gain weight over time, so don't be too quick to blame all weight gain on quitting or to use it as an excuse to return to smoking. Most of the weight gained more than six months after quitting is probably not due to having stopped smoking. If you find your weight is creeping outside of your comfort zone, you may wish to revisit Chapters 3 and 4 to reinforce the weight-management skills you've been cultivating.

YOUR PERSONAL STYLE

Over the years, consciously or unconsciously, you have created and developed your own personal style. What you wear—your taste in clothes—is part of it. So is your makeup, your hairstyle, how you decorate your home, the way you walk and talk. But it is more than that—it is some combination of all these things that represents your attitude toward the world, how you project your personality, your approach to life. It is how you maximize your strengths and minimize your weaknesses. If you scrutinize your favorite actresses and models closely, you will see that none of them is perfect. They all have flaws—a mouth too big, hips too wide, a waist too thick. But they have learned to distract attention away from these features or even to turn them into assets, as part of their unique "signature."

If you are a smoker, then that, too, has become part of your personal style. Your cigarettes have become an extension of your body; they say something about how you carry yourself and move; they are part of how you express yourself.

Part of the challenge, and also the joy, of quitting smoking will be adjusting your personal style to accommodate your new nonsmoking status. On the most elementary level, this means finding something else to do with your hands and mouth during the times you used to spend smoking, as discussed above. But more than that, it means maximizing the strengths associated with being a nonsmoker and minimizing anything that seems to you to be a flaw. It means moving through life with confidence and poise. It means feeling, as the French say, *bien dans ta peau*—"comfortable in your skin."

Moving through life without cigarettes will probably seem awkward at first. This is hardly surprising—considering that if you smoke a pack a day, you move your hand to your lips, inhale, and then blow out a cloud of smoke approximately two hundred times each and every day. You may need to make a conscious effort to get beyond the inevitable feeling that something is missing, that you're not quite at home in your world. Here are a few suggestions to get you started.

* Once your body size and shape have stabilized, use some of the money you saved by not buying cigarettes to purchase some new clothes that flatter you as you are now, confident that they will look and smell fresh and clean as they never did when you were a smoker. Put your cigarette money in a glass jar so you can see it accumulate. Shop when you have plenty of time to try on lots of styles and colors. Vertical stripes, darker hues, A-line shapes— these are all supposed to be slimming, but you'll need some quality fitting room time to find out what really works for you. Above all, wear clothes that fit. Clothing that is neither too tight nor too baggy looks best on most of us. If you can't stand the idea of being a size 12 instead of a 10, cut the label out!

* Get your hair restyled, confident that it will no longer reek of tobacco.

* Get your teeth cleaned and whitened, confident that they will stay that way.

* If polished and well-shaped nails are "you," get a manicure, confident that your nails and fingertips will look better now that you're no longer smoking.

* Treat yourself to a facial, confident that you've slowed down the wrinkling process by quitting.

* Give someone special a hug, confident that you don't reek of tobacco smoke.

* Gather some flowers from your yard or buy a small bouquet, enjoying the fragrance more than you have since you began smoking.

* Pay a little extra attention to your posture. Look at your body in a mirror and notice the difference that standing up straight or hunching over makes. Suck in your abs and hold your chin up! Amazingly, how you stand and hold your body can add pounds to or subtract pounds from how you look. (Once again, your mother was right!)

Once you get going, you'll undoubtedly come up with additional ideas that are particularly well-matched to your own personal style.

6

Special Concerns

As if dealing with eating and exercise weren't enough, many women have additional challenges to face when they stop smoking. This chapter deals with some of the circumstances women are likely to encounter, including relationship problems, issues relating to pregnancy and postpartum, obesity, large weight gain, eating disorders, and depression. Feel free to skip over the sections that don't apply to you and jump right to those that do.

RELATIONSHIP ISSUES

Change—whether it be quitting smoking or eating differently or starting a fitness program—doesn't occur in a vacuum. Change, even for the better, affects not just the person making the change but also her interactions with family and friends. "Social support" and encouragement from those you love can be extremely helpful, especially if you are skilled in mobilizing it. A spouse who openly takes pride in your accomplishments, compliments your efforts, or offers to care for the kids while you go to the gym can provide a tremendous boost. Not everyone is so fortunate, however, and family members may intentionally or unintentionally make it harder for you to carry out your commitment to change by criticizing or expressing dissatisfaction.

When Your Partner or Family Sabotages Your Efforts to Change Your Eating Patterns or Avoid Weight Gain

What about the partner who is threatened by the changes you are making in your eating, exercise, and smoking patterns and subtly (or perhaps not so subtly) undermines your efforts? Clinicians call this well-known phenomenon "sabotage," and it can take many forms. Here are few examples:

"Try these doughnuts I made."

"It's no fun eating when you nibble on that rabbit food."

"Aren't you ever going to be done with that diet?"

"Please help me finish this dessert."

"That damn treadmill drowns out the TV. Wouldn't it be more fun to curl up together on the sofa?"

"Let's go out on the porch and have a cigarette together."

The infrastructure of intimate relationships is often made up less of shared philosophies and big ideas than of shared daily routines like eating, watching television…and smoking. There is nothing wrong with this *per se*. We all become comfortable with these patterns, and it is disruptive if one person wants to change and the other doesn't. Moreover, your partner may secretly welcome your lapses because they reinforce his or her conviction that it is too difficult to stop overeating, under-exercising, or smoking; your slips may ease your partner's guilt, anxiety, or feelings of weakness associated with persisting in these patterns.

So how do you deal with this situation? You can start by reassuring your partner that the changes you are making do not signal any change in your fundamental relationship. You can plan nonfood-related activities to compensate for the loss of the mealtime camaraderie associated with eating the same dish or sharing dessert. You can try to schedule your exercise sessions so they don't take away from the time you spend together. You can convey your appreciation for any expression of support, however stingy. You can come right out and ask for his or her help, emphasizing how much it would mean to you. Try to keep things low-key and avoid confrontations that can have no good resolution. Professional counseling may be an option if your partner is agreeable.

If all these gambits fail, you may be forced to tune out the complaints and blandishments, trusting that eventually your partner will come around. Distasteful as this may be, and contrary to your usual mode of interacting, this situation is preferable to feeling miserable in your skin or despising yourself and your body. It will also make you more pleasant to be around—even if your partner is unaware of being the chief beneficiary of your commitment to maintaining self- and life-affirming behavior patterns!

When Your Partner Is Overly Invested in Controlling Your Weight

Shelley, an acquaintance of mine, once went for a drive in the countryside with her husband, Jim. When Shelley reached for a snack, Jim, a private pilot, remarked, "Food can't fly past your eyes without making a landing in your mouth." Although she laughed about it later, at the time she felt very angry and hurt; she was angry that he was policing her food intake and hurt because the subtext was clear: "You're too fat."

Some partners adopt the role of "food cop" or "exercise cop," either for weight or health reasons. They may pride themselves on their superior willpower or restraint and judge you if you fall short of their standards. They may scold you for eating certain foods and ask about what you ate when you were out. They may probe into when you last went to the gym.

These expressions are often well intended, and, assuming there is underlying goodwill in the relationship, the problem can generally be confronted directly, by making your partner more aware of these acts and their impact on you. Point out that you need to take ownership of your weight-management program and can only be responsible for your successes if you're also responsible for your slips. Try reverse role-playing so that your partner can experience the effects of having one's personal behavior so closely monitored and scrutinized.

At the extreme other end of the spectrum from the saboteur is the partner who goes beyond policing and exerts strong pressure on you to be thin—even if you are not seriously overweight to begin with. This pressure may surprise you by emerging only after you gain a few pounds. Or you may have even been attracted to his obsession with thinness. The writer Molly Jong-Fast, for example, describes her involvement with a man who "decided he might be able to love me if I was a size 6." When she reached this goal, he told her she'd look even better if she were a size 4.

Sadly, a few men (and these thinness connoisseurs tend to be men) are so invested in their partners' appearance that they view any increase in weight as little short of a breach of contract—even if they themselves have piled on the pounds since the honeymoon! There's a fine line between being supportive of your efforts or complimentary of the results or concerned about your health, on the one hand, and implying, on the other hand, that his affection is linked with your appearance and subject to being withheld if you don't meet certain standards. It is a fine line, but a critically important one. The latter is totally inappropriate.

Allowing a misguided partner to seize control of your feelings about your body is not consistent with the goal of taking charge of your life and will not help you feel good about yourself. If your own weight concerns are driven not from within but by partner pressures or fears of withdrawal of affection, first be sure that these attitudes are not something that you are projecting onto your partner but truly emanate from him. If, after discussion and reflection, you determine that the messages about thinness are indeed coming from him, and that he prioritizes your being thin over your quitting smoking, then it is likely that your relationship has serious fault lines, and professional counseling may be required. If your partner won't go, then go by yourself.

PREGNANCY AND POSTPARTUM

A special case of the weight-concerned smoker is the pregnant smoker, or the smoker who anticipates becoming pregnant. When women smokers become pregnant, they are asked to control weight gain and at the same time to relinquish an addictive drug with weight-suppressing effects, while watching their bodies balloon. As my colleagues and I at the Nicotine Research Laboratory found in a study of women who had given birth to their first child within the past ten years and were smokers at the time that they became pregnant, women who have been using smoking as a tool for managing weight may actually end up gaining *excessive* weight during pregnancy.

Virtually nothing you can do for the baby you're expecting is more positive than quitting smoking prior to becoming pregnant or as soon as you learn that you're pregnant. But if in addition to quitting you can manage your weight during pregnancy, you'll feel better about yourself and be less likely to resume smoking during the pregnancy or after delivery. Staying within the targets set by the Institute of Medicine will make it easier to recover your prepregnancy weight than if you exceed the guidelines. Recommended weight gain is as follows: 28 to 40 pounds if you were *underweight* prior to pregnancy, 25 to 35 pounds if you were *normal weight*, 15 to 25 pounds if you were *overweight*, and 11 to 20 pounds if you were *obese*.

Most of the suggestions I've offered for controlling food intake apply to pregnant women as well. Unless you are carrying twins or multiples, the average pregnant woman should eat about three hundred additional calories per day—*assuming she is not overeating to begin with*. If you are quitting smoking, ask your obstetrician or midwife if you can limit your increase in food intake to one hundred to two hundred calories per day to offset possible postcessation increases in weight.

Similarly, most of my suggestions for increasing physical activity can be easily adapted to the needs of the pregnant woman. The American College of Obstetricians and Gynecologists encourages pregnant women to exercise thirty minutes per day. Most advisable restrictions and modifications are commonsense: Concentrate on low-impact forms of exercise, avoid inversions and other extreme yoga positions, and do not exercise in an overheated room or sauna. Take frequent breaks and drink lots of water. Do not engage in exercise that requires lying on your back after the first trimester.

An alternative approach that's okay with some pregnant women is to give yourself permission to gain a little extra weight at a time when it is "bundled" with the socially acceptable weight gain that goes with pregnancy. After all, most women, smokers or not, expect to have to work on their weight a little bit once the baby is born. Don't go overboard, though. The idea is to tolerate a small amount of weight gain after quitting in the context of a healthful prenatal nutritional pattern; it is not a time to abandon moderation altogether. The last thing you need as a new mom and former smoker, as we'll see in the next section, is a lot of stubborn excess weight to shed.

After the Baby Arrives

The first few weeks after a baby is born are a particularly difficult time for women who have quit smoking during their pregnancy. You're exhausted and overwhelmed with your new responsibilities. You may even have a case of the "postpartum blues." Unless you're breastfeeding, you've been given the green light to resume use of caffeine and alcohol—activities that in the past have often occurred in conjunction with smoking. When you look in the mirror, it strikes home that not all the weight you gained during pregnancy is accounted for by the weight of the baby. If you're planning to return to work, you may be concerned about fitting into your "grown-up clothes." Especially if quitting was motivated primarily by a desire to protect your unborn child, it may be tempting to return to the old comforts of smoking.

As you've undoubtedly heard, exposure to environmental tobacco smoke and, if you're nursing, to nicotine in breast milk, is not the best thing for your baby, so the need to protect your child doesn't end with delivery. But it is not just about your baby; it is also about you—and protecting the investment you've made in quitting already. The first few days of abstaining are the hardest; do you really want to go through that again?

It is normal for it to take several weeks or even months to get back to your prepregnancy weight. If you're breastfeeding, the last few pounds may not drop off until the baby is weaned. Try to take pleasure and pride in your body and the amazing feat it has just accomplished. If you've ever wished for larger breasts, enjoy your new voluptuous figure.

Now that your body is your own again, take time to review

and renew the self-coaching skills you developed in Chapters 2 through 5. The best thing you can do for yourself is to take an active role in the process of restoring your body to the shape and size that feels right to you.

Having a baby—especially your first—is a major life change, one that means reinventing yourself as a mom and reconciling the image of the attractive woman you want to be with that of someone who also changes diapers and mops up spit-up milk (and worse). This is definitely a challenge! But it is one that many women have met with grace and charm. So can you. And doing it as a nonsmoker will help you feel good about both yourself and your baby.

Note: As we will see in later in the chapter, smoking and depression often go hand in hand. The fact that you have been a smoker *may* mean that you are a person who is prone to depression. During and after pregnancy are times of intense hormonal, physical, and social role change that can upend the lives of even the most laid-back women. If you find that you are seriously depressed or are having a difficult time coming to terms with being a mother, *please* don't try to go it alone. There is great personal strength in knowing when to ask for help. Your health-care provider or religious leader should be able to support you in getting your life back on track without your resorting to smoking or to refer you to someone who can.

OBESITY

So far we have talked mostly about women whose main problem is that they don't want to gain weight when they quit. They are either satisfied with their current weight or perhaps somewhat dissatisfied, but in any event they can't face the prospect—in addition to that of giving up their cigarettes— of feeling worse about their bodies and themselves. Calling these "cosmetic" reasons does not do justice to the dilemma these women face, so I generally try to avoid that word. As I have said repeatedly, unless these reasons are taken seriously and addressed straightforwardly, we will leave thousands of women smokers lost in an impossible psychic Bermuda Triangle, where they can't get right with themselves no matter what they do.

There is another category of woman smoker, however, whose weight-related concerns also need to be addressed, and that is the woman smoker who is medically overweight or obese to begin with. The weight crisis in the United States has now reached epidemic proportions, with approximately one-third of the population qualifying as "obese," and an additional one-third as "medically overweight." You may find it hard to accept the idea that a condition occurring in more than half the population is not defined as "normal." But this is not a case of "all the children are above average," as in Garrison Keillor's Lake Wobegon. Desirable weight ranges can be determined objectively by relating them statistically to health outcomes, and as Americans we are now collectively wandering into a danger zone in which a large proportion of us are exposing ourselves to the health risks associated with excess weight.

Despite the weight-suppressing effects of nicotine, smokers have by no means escaped the obesity epidemic. Of the nearly one thousand women smokers who have participated in our studies, 24 percent are obese, and another 26 percent are medically overweight. Many of these women probably have additional health problems associated with smoking, obesity, or both, including diabetes, elevated cholesterol, and high blood pressure. For health reasons, these women cannot afford to gain weight, but they also cannot afford to continue smoking.

Are You Medically Overweight?

Do you think you may fall into this category? In the Nicotine Research Laboratory, we distinguish among three different concepts of body weight and shape: (1) how you really look, (2) how you *think* you really look, and (3) how you would *like* to look. The difference between the first and second conceptualizations is an index of body image; if the difference is very large, then you probably have a distorted body image. ("Body image" is a complex concept that refers to perceptions about the body, particularly but not exclusively focused on appearance. A person of normal weight who sees a very fat person in the mirror has a distorted body image—and possibly a psychiatric condition called "body dysmorphic disorder.") At least some degree of distortion is not uncommon; in a recent survey of college women, 75 percent of those who described themselves as "too fat" were actually of normal weight, and 5 percent were clinically underweight. The third conceptualization could be construed as your goal; if the difference between the first and third conceptualizations is very large, then you may have unrealistic expectations, which is a formula for misery since you can never be satisfied. (We could probably add a fourth conceptualization: the highest weight you could live with and still feel okay about yourself.)

The first of these conceptualizations, however, is the only one that is completely objective and linked to your actual body weight and shape (and to your physical health). For the purposes of this chapter, then, *overweight* and *obese* will be defined in terms of the indicator used by the National Institutes of Health and by most researchers, the body mass index (BMI), sometimes referred to as the Quetelet Index. BMI is basically an index of weight *corrected for height*. Intuitively, this should make sense. You and your friend may both weigh 160 pounds, for example, but if you are five feet tall, and she's six feet tall, she is at a desirable weight, but you are obese.

What's your BMI? There are a number of BMI calculators and tables available on the Web, including the site for the new government dietary guidelines (www.cdc.gov/healthyweight/assessing/bmi/). The formula for BMI is given in the metric system—[weight in kilograms] divided by [height in meters squared]—but a close approximation can be quite easily computed with a hand calculator, or even (horrors!) using arithmetic, using the following formula:

1. Multiply your weight in pounds by 703: _____.

2. Multiply your height in inches by your height in inches (in other words, your height squared): _____.

3. Divide the answer you get in step 1 by the answer you get in step 2: _____. This is your BMI.

If your answer isn't somewhere between 15 and 60—and more likely between 18 and 40—you probably made a mistake in your calculations. Go back and try again.

The BMI has some limitations. It doesn't take into account variations in body build. It may overestimate body fat in elite athletes and individuals with a very muscular build. It may underestimate body fat in older people and individuals who have lost muscle mass because of illness or extreme inactivity. For most people, however—including almost all women—it is a good approximation of how lean or fat you are.

In addition, waist size is sometimes used as an index of abdominal fat, with a waist size of 35 inches or more considered to be undesirable in women. Because smoking affects fat deposition, however, quitting may affect your waist size independently of your body weight, so I recommend calculating and using your BMI as your guide.

So...now (ta-DAH!) we are ready to answer the question of whether you are medically overweight. Here are the official guidelines for adults, and the ones we will use in this book:

* If your BMI is below 18.5, you are underweight.
* If your BMI is between 18.5 and 24.9, you are of normal weight.
* If your BMI is between 25.0 and 29.9, you are overweight.
* If your BMI is 30.0 or higher, you are obese.

Important: This is not the same as how you might describe or feel about your weight. If you have a BMI of 24.5, you may well think you'd look better if you lost weight. You might even be at a slightly more desirable weight from a health point of view if you lost a little weight (or maybe not; the jury's still out on this question). But the overall health risks of having a BMI below 25 are minimal. You are not "overweight" as defined by health-related criteria; you are not *medically* overweight.

If you are medically overweight but not obese, you are in a bit of a gray zone, health-wise. National Institute of Health guidelines suggest that you may not be at excessive health risk unless you have at least two additional risk factors. By defini-tion, you have one risk factor if you are a smoker. Other risk factors include:

* high blood pressure (hypertension)
* high LDL cholesterol (low-density lipoprotein, or "bad" cholesterol)
* low HDL cholesterol (high-density lipoprotein, or "good" cholesterol)
* high triglycerides
* high blood glucose (sugar)
* family history of premature heart disease
* physical inactivity

If you have no risk factor other than smoking, then maintaining your weight is generally regarded as an acceptable health outcome. But here's the catch: Eliminating smoking (and that's why you're reading this book, isn't it?) may make it harder to maintain your weight. Moreover, if you have two additional risk factors, theoretically you should not only be maintaining weight, you should be losing it.

If you are in the "obese" category, your weight poses a health risk regardless of other factors. Certainly you should do whatever you can to minimize weight gain when you quit smoking. And here there's actually a bit of good news: The higher your initial body weight, on average, the less weight you are likely to gain when you quit smoking.

That being said, most experts would probably agree that a *modest* weight gain is an acceptable health tradeoff for stopping smoking. In fact, to the extent that the increase in overweight in our country represents a decline in smoking, it can't be regarded as an unqualified negative.

What constitutes a modest weight gain? One way of looking at it is that each unit increase in BMI represents about five to seven pounds (five pounds if you are five feet tall, seven if you're six feet). If you can avoid increasing your BMI by more than one unit, and if you can avoid going into a higher-risk category than you are already in (that is, from "normal weight" to "overweight," or "overweight" to "obese"), then strictly from a health perspective your postcessation weight gain would not be regarded as excessive when compared with the health benefits of quitting smoking.

So in short, the recommendations provided in Chapters 3 to 5 of this book are no different from those you would follow if you were in the normal weight range. If you are already medically overweight or obese, however, some additional caveats are required, considerations to which you should pay attention in deference to your physical health:

1. Check with your health-care provider before undertaking an exercise program.

2. If you have not had a complete physical examination recently, do so in order to rule out metabolic disorders such as thyroid disease that might contribute to your excess weight.

If postcessation weight gain cannot be controlled using the measures described above, please seek additional help *promptly*. Again, check with your health-care provider. In extreme instances, prescription medications or bariatric surgery may be indicated. And, of course, see the "Additional Reading and Resources for Weight and Mood Management" section at the end of this book.

LARGE WEIGHT GAIN

A few women—a little less than 15 percent—gain in excess of thirty pounds when they quit smoking. One woman, for example, told us she'd gained one hundred pounds during a previous attempt to quit. Many (though not all) of these large gainers probably have clinical or subclinical eating disorders, such as binge-eating disorder, which they have been "medicating" with nicotine. Others may be overeating in response to depression, which sometimes emerges following smoking cessation. Still others may have metabolic conditions, as yet unexplained, that emerge or reemerge when no longer held in check by nicotine.

Even if they are not medically overweight or obese to begin with, women who gain large amounts of weight when they quit smoking are at risk of ending up in the "danger zone" in which postcessation weight gain constitutes a serious health risk. This means creeping into the medically "overweight" (BMI between 25 and 29.9) or "obese" (BMI of 30 or above) ranges. To determine your personal cutoffs for these categories, do the following:

1. Multiply your height in inches by your height in inches (in other words, your height squared): _____.
2. Multiply the answer you get in step 1 by 25: _____.
3. Divide the answer you get in step 2 by 703: _____. If this were your weight, you'd have a BMI of 25.

Now determine the weight you would be if you had a BMI of 30: Repeat the above procedure except that in step 2, multiply the answer in step 1 by 30. To have a BMI of 30, your weight would have to be _____.

If, a few weeks after quitting, you find that your weight, previously normal, is approaching either of these cutoffs—because you are unable to carry out the measures recommended in Chapters 3 and 4 or in spite of carrying them out—then a more intensive intervention may be needed. After all the work you've invested in quitting, *please* do not return to smoking. Like the smoker who was medically overweight or obese to begin with, however, you should seek help promptly from your health-care provider or check out the "Additional Reading and Resources for Weight and Mood Management" section in the back of the book. Finally, read ahead to the next two sections if you suspect your excessive weight gain is related to an eating disorder or depression.

DISORDERED EATING

Many smokers have quit in response to extensive public health campaigns and the availability of medications that improve the chances of success. By studying those who nevertheless continue to smoke, researchers have determined that certain groups of people are at increased risk of starting to smoke in the first place and are likely to have difficulties in quitting. For example, depressed people, and even those with a history of depression, are about twice as likely to be smokers as people without such a history. Similarly, people with diagnosable or subclinical eating disorders are more likely to smoke than people without these conditions. Because disordered eating (and the body image problems that often accompany it) and depression are so common among women, this section and the one that follows will focus on these conditions and their potential for undermining how you look and feel in the context of quitting smoking.

When we first became interested in studying "weight-control smoking" at the Nicotine Research Laboratory, we quickly discovered that women who endorsed smoking as a method for controlling weight also scored higher on measures of both restrained or restrictive eating (dieting) and disinhibited or unrestrained eating (binge eating).

Cotinine is a breakdown product of nicotine in the human body. Its concentration in the bloodstream can give you an idea of how much someone smokes. The more you smoke, the more you're exposed to nicotine's weight-suppressing effects, so that the higher the cotinine levels, the lower the smoker's weight, on average, would be expected to be. Well, that's exactly what we found—but *only* in those smokers who did not endorse "weight-control smoking." The relationship between weight and cotinine levels was much less pronounced in weight-control smokers, suggesting that these smokers were not *just* using smoking to control their weight but also adding other methods, such as restrictive eating, to the mix.

What we came to suspect is that at least some of our weight-control smokers were "using" nicotine to manage a tendency toward binge eating. This hunch led us to delve deeper into the link between smoking and eating disorders. Our first study involved a re-analysis of data collected by Dr. Dean Krahn, an expert in eating disorders, in women just before they began their first year at the University of Michigan. Krahn had given these young women a questionnaire that included items designed to assess dieting and binge-eating behavior in college students, as well as a variety of questions about lifestyle and drug use. He originally presented his data based on dieting categories, but when we reorganized his data so that we could make comparisons based on smoking status, we found considerably more dieting and other unhealthful eating practices in the smokers than in the nonsmokers.

Well, we all know that serious eating disorders are primarily a young woman's health problem, don't we? Or do we? Actually, the extent to which these patterns persist into later adulthood is not well understood. So we started giving the same questionnaire to adult smokers who participated in studies at the Nicotine Research Laboratory, and although the data were not quite so dramatic as those provided by the college student smokers, nearly 15 percent were classified as being "at risk," and 4 percent gave responses consistent with a clinical diagnosis of an eating disorder. We subsequently confirmed, in a national random sample of women, that smokers scored higher than never-smokers on this scale, on average, and were more likely to have scores indicative of eating disorders.

We believe that when these women stop smoking, binge eating may reemerge in full force. As noted above, in our discussion of large weight gain, these are the women we expect will end up gaining weight in amounts that, unlike normal weight gain after quitting smoking, may actually be dangerous to their health.

An eating binge is technically defined as eating a larger amount of food than normal over, say, a two-hour period. During this episode, the person feels a lack of control over eating. Other characteristics associated with binge eating are eating until uncomfortably full; eating when not hungry; eating rapidly; eating alone or in secret; or feeling guilt, shame, or disgust about eating. Almost everyone overeats occasionally; pigging out at Thanksgiving does not qualify as an eating disorder. But if you find yourself going on an eating binge a couple of times a week, you may be suffering from binge-eating disorder.

If you have any suspicion that you have binge-eating disorder, be kind to yourself and seek professional help. There are excellent therapists who specialize in eating disorders who can help you overcome this persistent problem. It will increase your chances of both quitting smoking and managing your weight; it will help you make peace with your own body.

Other eating disorders include anorexia nervosa and bulimia nervosa. Anorexia, the eating disorder that makes the most headlines, is not particularly associated with smoking. Anorexics have a body weight that is 15 percent below normal weight in the absence of an underlying medical condition, and often they do not menstruate. Weight loss is achieved by fasting, excessive exercise, chewing food and spitting it out, and/or so-called compensatory behaviors (purging, either by self-induced vomiting or using laxatives). Individuals with bulimia, by contrast, are usually of normal weight. Bulimia is typically characterized by cycles of binge eating followed by purging. Bulimia is overrepresented among smokers. Indeed, I have sometimes entertained the thought that for some women, smoking should be classified as a compensatory behavior.

Many psychiatrists, by the way, see eating disorders as a form of addiction. Like other addictions, it frequently goes hand in hand with depression and with other substance use. Because it often occurs in secret, and because weight loss is often praised until it becomes excessive, it is difficult to detect. Because—unlike drug use—eating is essential to life, it can be especially difficult to treat. Great strides have been made in recent years in the treatment of eating disorders, however, and there is a lot more help available today.

The behaviors described above must occur fairly frequently to meet diagnostic criteria, and true anorexia and bulimia are therefore relatively uncommon. Many women, however, flirt with these behaviors at some time in their lives, and a fair number of women have eating patterns that, while falling short of a full-blown eating-disorders diagnosis, are potentially dangerous. Engaging in purging is never "normal" and should not be shrugged off. If you find yourself tempted to control weight via these dangerous behaviors, again, I urge you to seek professional help—ideally from a team that includes a therapist, a dietitian, and a medical doctor. Hospitalization may be required if the binge/purge cycle is severe enough to affect physical health.

DEPRESSION

Why talk about depression in a book about smoking and how you look? First of all, it is hard to look your best if you're feeling miserable and blue. The smile on your face and the spring in your step disappear, and your slumping posture radiates dejection. Second, depression often makes it much harder to do the things you need to do to manage your weight—namely, eating mindfully and exercising mindfully. It undermines your motivation to take care of yourself and erodes your sense of your personal style.

Of all the psychological conditions associated with smoking, depression is the most extensively documented. As noted above, whether it is clinically diagnosed or measured on scales developed to evaluate people in the community, depression is more common in smokers than in nonsmokers. The reasons for this association are not clearly understood, though there is some evidence to support the idea that smoking enhances mood and represents a form of self-medication.

What are the implications for quitting? Depressed mood is part of the "official" tobacco withdrawal syndrome, along with anxiety and difficulty concentrating. But it is a relatively rare symptom, occurring in only approximately one in five quitters. And unlike other withdrawal symptoms, it is rather consistently associated with relapse to smoking.

Is it possible that people with a history of depression are particularly likely to experience depressed mood as a withdrawal symptom? To answer this question, my colleagues and I at the Nicotine Research Laboratory studied 365 smokers who provided data on the withdrawal symptoms they experienced during past attempts to quit, as well as on measures of depression and other psychological conditions. Sure enough, we found that depressed mood as a withdrawal symptom did not occur randomly but was much more likely to occur in people who scored high on our measure of depression.

We subsequently confirmed this observation in a quitting study in which women were divided into groups by whether they had high or low scores on depression prior to quitting. The women who started with low depression scores showed only a mild elevation in depressed mood during the first week that leveled off during the second week. By contrast, women who started with scores consistent with clinical depression showed depression scores that were markedly elevated in the first week and continued to climb in the second week.

We have not studied smoking cessation in patients in treatment for depression in the Nicotine Research Laboratory, but colleagues who have have reported occasional instances of a full-blown depressive episode when these patients quit smoking. The depression generally resolves if they resume smoking—but depression is a treatable condition, and seeking an effective treatment is a more appropriate response than resuming smoking.

Everyone has ups and downs, even under the best of circumstances, and a certain amount of moodiness is normal when you first quit smoking. True depression generally persists for at least two weeks. Although it often involves feeling extremely blue and down-in-the-dumps, it may also manifest itself as a profound lack of energy and loss of interest in the things that normally give you pleasure. Other symptoms of depression include persistent inability to sleep or excessive sleeping, fatigue, feelings of emptiness or uselessness, recurrent thoughts of death or suicide, inability to concentrate, indecisiveness, and change in appetite or weight (either decrease or increase) when not dieting (or quitting smoking). Depression may also manifest itself via physical symptoms such as headache or stomach upset. Problems at work and excessive alcohol use may be associated with depression.

Have you ever been diagnosed with depression, or do you think you might be clinically depressed right now? Don't let this deter you from thinking about quitting smoking, but please remain alert for signs of trouble when you quit, and be quick to seek professional help if you start experiencing exaggerated feelings of hopelessness or despair. It is an act of strength, not weakness, to ask for help when you need it. Your family doctor or health practitioner can help you.

I also encourage you to consider using a stop-smoking

medication. Unless you are a very light smoker, nicotine replacement products are an option for you. You should ask your health-care provider about Zyban. As noted above, Zyban is also marketed as Wellbutrin, an antidepressant. If your insurance policy doesn't cover smoking-cessation medications, ask your doctor if you might be a candidate for Wellbutrin instead; it is the same drug. Recently, it has become available in generic form under the name bupropion, which is more affordable than the name-brand product.

For people with less-severe forms of depressed mood, such as may occur following smoking cessation, the following tips may be helpful:

* Don't forget about the mood-brightening effects of exercise, as described in Chapter 4. Aerobic exercise in amounts recommended by government guidelines has been shown to be an effective treatment for mild-to-moderate depression.

* Another depression-buster may be snuggling with your partner, your children, or your pet. Really! Loving contact and even loving thoughts can trigger the release of oxytocin, the hormone that stimulates uterine contraction during labor and milk release during nursing. There is also evidence to suggest that it plays a role in maternal caregiving and pair-bonding after puberty. Experts call this "affiliative behavior," and disruptions such as relationship problems often characterize depression in women. Even if this theory falls by the wayside, isn't it a great prescription?

* Some people seem to be born happy. But even if you're not among them, many people find it possible to *learn* to be happier by finding ways to "jolly themselves up," whether by distracting themselves or "thought-stopping" when sad

or worrisome thoughts intrude, by exercising, by schooling themselves to avoid self-blame, by spending more time socializing with others, or by engaging in some pleasurable activity. Sometimes if you *act* happy, the emotions will obediently fall into line behind the behavior. Even the simple act of smiling can lift your spirits. Try it and see. (It goes without saying, of course, that comforting yourself by gorging on food is not such a good idea and, once the eating stops, leaves you feeling worse, not better.)

If you notice symptoms of depression, including overeating and weight gain, that are largely confined to the fall or winter months, you may be suffering from a form of depression called seasonal affective disorder (SAD). In its most severe form, SAD may require professional intervention and medication. Up to 20 percent of Americans may suffer from milder forms of SAD, however, with women making up the majority of this number. These people can often benefit from additional exposure to the sun (and if you get it by taking long walks outdoors, so much the better!) Also helpful is light therapy or phototherapy, which involves exposure to light from a special fluorescent lamp a few hours per day during the winter months.

At least one study has demonstrated a positive effect of light exposure in nonseasonal depression, and an exploratory trial suggests it may also be effective for depression during pregnancy. I have often wondered whether phototherapy might be helpful in promoting smoking cessation, especially for those 20 percent of individuals who experience depressed mood as a smoking withdrawal symptom. I never had the opportunity to test this hypothesis, so I have no scientific evidence that it will be helpful. At this point, it is in the category of "can't hurt, might help."

7

Quitting for Good

As I said early on, this book is not intended as a how-to-quit manual *per se*. The focus is on helping women who have smoked, whether now or in the past, become more comfortable with their post-smoking selves and bodies. Along the way, I've offered many suggestions to keep you looking and feeling great without any "help" from that false friend, the cigarette. Some of these hints and pointers are similar to those a traditional smoking-cessation counselor would offer; others go beyond, drawing on my own experiences with women smokers who want to quit but are also deeply concerned about what will happen when they do. All of this information should contribute to helping you quit and stay quit by making you, not cigarettes, the boss of your body.

We've almost reached the end of our journey, and if you're already a confirmed former smoker, you may prefer to skip ahead to the final chapter to hear the rest of the good news about life after cigarettes. Or perhaps you're among the fortunate few who can wake up one day, decide they've had it with smoking, and throw out all their cigarettes without fishing them out of the trash a few hours later.

But if you haven't yet quit—or if, like Mark Twain, you've found that quitting smoking is easy ("I know because I've done it thousands of times") but staying quit is another story—you may feel the need for a summary of the recommendations on quitting scattered throughout this book, along with guidance on other issues that aren't directly covered. This chapter is for you.

WHY IT IS SO HARD TO QUIT

Let's first take a moment to unpack smoking and nicotine dependence. As I've already noted, if you smoke a pack a day and take 10 puffs on each cigarette, that's 200 puffs each day and nearly 75,000 puffs each year. Even if you smoke "only" half a pack, that's over 35,000 puffs a year. It is hard to think of any other voluntary activity (be it something you have to do or something you like to do) that you do so often. This very frequency creates many, many opportunities for pairing the act of smoking with other staples of your daily life—driving, sorting the mail, watching television, waiting "on hold" on the phone, or sharing a cup of coffee with a friend. When you start going about your business without a cigarette in your hands, it is no wonder you feel as though something is missing.

Of course, you wouldn't have gotten into this vicious cycle if cigarettes were made from lettuce leaves. Nicotine, the principal psychoactive ingredient in tobacco, has stimulant, antianxiety, antipain, and antidepressant effects when delivered rapidly to the brain. The cigarette is perfectly designed for doing just that: With each puff, nicotine is absorbed in the lung, enters the bloodstream, and reaches the brain in approximately seven seconds. The effects may not knock you off your feet, but they are reliable and available on demand. Since you've probably been smoking since long before you reached the age of consent, if you're like most smokers, you've learned that you can count on your cigarette to give you a little lift if you're feeling blue, wake you up if you're feeling drowsy, or calm you down if you're feeling anxious.

The nicotine molecule has a shape that enables it to bind to receptors for the neurotransmitter acetylcholine, which is involved in many basic life functions including muscle movement, breathing, learning, memory, and as we saw in Chapter 2, metabolic processes. When nicotine enters the brain, it attaches itself to receptors in reward pathways, initiating a cascade of effects that include the release of dopamine, a neurotransmitter that affects emotional response and ability to experience pleasure and pain. These pathways evolved to protect us by motivating us to do what we need to survive both as individuals and as a species. Nicotine delivered via inhaled smoke, by mimicking acetylcholine, essentially hijacks these systems, providing pleasure, elevating mood, and relieving anxiety in ways that Mother Nature decidedly never intended. These favorable effects increase the likelihood that we will repeat the behavior that produced them—namely, smoking. There is good evidence from our laboratory and those of others to suggest that people who go on to become addicted smokers are particularly sensitive to the pleasurable effects of smoking when they first experiment with tobacco as teenagers (even if they also experience unpleasant sensations such as nausea). We have also published a report suggesting a genetic basis for this initial sensitivity.

With repeated exposure, the receptors activated by nicotine adapt by becoming less sensitive, leading to the phenomenon known as tolerance—that is, more drug is needed to produce the same effect. If you stop smoking abruptly, the unoccupied receptors "miss" their expected dose of nicotine, producing a characteristic withdrawal syndrome that in addition to increased appetite, weight gain, and depressed mood—already covered at length in this book—is likely to include some or all of the following:

* anxiety

* irritability, frustration, or anger

* difficulty concentrating

* sleep disturbances

* restlessness

Tolerance and withdrawal are traditionally the hallmarks of any form of drug dependence, including nicotine dependence.

Are you dependent (or addicted—I'll use the terms interchangeably here)? Although there are schemes for categorizing individuals as dependent or nondependent smokers, tobacco dependence is probably best conceptualized as a continuum ranging from little or no dependence to a high level of dependence. If you smoke your first cigarette of the day within thirty minutes of waking, if you smoke a pack or more per day, if you crave cigarettes when they're not available or have trouble keeping from smoking when it is not allowed, then you're highly dependent. Many women smoke only ten cigarettes per day, however, and still show signs of being dependent smokers. In fact, in susceptible individuals, dependence can develop quite rapidly after initial exposure, as evidenced by the many young adolescents who, having started, find it is not nearly as easy to stop as they'd expected.

As we noted in Chapter 2, there are a few women who may truly be termed "social smokers." Many are college students who are using their newfound freedom to experiment with tobacco. They may smoke on Friday night in a bar or occasionally light up in a dorm room with friends, but they do not smoke on a daily basis. They may or may not inhale. They are probably minimally dependent on nicotine, if at all. If you are a social smoker, here are two things you should know:

1. You probably won't gain weight when you quit because you

aren't using nicotine frequently enough or in large enough amounts to suppress weight or appetite in the first place.

2. You are flirting with becoming a dependent smoker.

Please stop smoking now while it is relatively easy to do so.

Most smokers, however, fall somewhere along the dependence continuum—that is, their behavior is at least to some extent unreasonably controlled by tobacco. They experience an urge or craving for a cigarette that can be measured as soon as a half hour after smoking, and that can persist for days, weeks, months, or even years after quitting. Unpleasant withdrawal symptoms also emerge, generally peaking within a few days but sometimes persisting much longer. Smoking a cigarette will quickly relieve craving and withdrawal—but sends the hapless would-be quitter back to square one. In surveys of illicit drug users, many endorse the belief that it would be more difficult to give up smoking than their drug of choice.

So don't be too hard on yourself if you're having trouble quitting, and don't be discouraged if you've tried unsuccessfully to quit in the past. Tobacco dependence is often referred to among clinicians as a chronic condition, in much the same way as diabetes and hypertension are chronic conditions, and the majority of those who quit make more than one attempt before they finally succeed. The fact that you haven't quit doesn't mean that you can't quit but rather that you haven't yet found the formula that matches best with your own "quitting style."

HOW YOU CAN QUIT

Throughout this book, I have tried to avoid advocating a single approach to change—whether it be a change in your eating patterns, your exercise routine, or your smoking behavior—but rather have tried to help you identify the approach or combination of approaches that will work best for you. An important premise of this book is that you know yourself better than anyone else could possibly know you. You're the world's expert on you, and you're in a better position than anyone else to determine what is likely to suit your needs. ***The best stop-smoking program for you is the one you can sustain over the long haul.***

This is not to suggest that all approaches are equally sound. If you Google "smoking cessation" or "quit smoking," you will find dozens of books, devices, herbal preparations, and procedures purporting to be miracle cures for smoking. A few are simply scams; others have been developed by individuals who are sincere in wanting to share with others what worked for them, however commonsensical or outrageous it may sound. Still others are treatments offered by legitimate practitioners (often accompanied by lavish testimonials to the effectiveness of their approach). Your cousin or your best friend from high school may swear by hypnosis or acupuncture, for example, and indeed, these methods appear to work for some people. In this book, however, I have focused on options based on or consistent with established clinical guidelines. These methods have survived the rigors of clinical testing in large numbers of smokers and are likely to be your best and safest bets. Fortunately, an extensive menu of trustworthy, evidence-based methods is available to help you quit smoking and stay quit, leaving you lots of latitude for choosing one that fits your general style and preference.

BEHAVIORAL TREATMENT OPTIONS

Ask yourself these questions: How do you generally approach the need to acquire new skills or make changes in your life? Do you learn better from self-help books, or would you rather use more interactive (and always available) methods such as you'll find on the Internet? Would you rather quit in a group setting, via telephone counseling, or one-on-one with a therapist?

In general, approaches involving either group or individual counseling have been shown to be more effective than self-help methods, treatments tailored to your specific needs are more effective than nonspecific treatment, and intensive interventions are more effective than minimal interventions. Still, if the idea of group treatment turns you off or you know from past experience that you aren't likely to stick with complex labor- and time-intensive methods, you're better off starting with something that more closely matches your preference.

Regardless of how minimal or intensive they might be, most behavioral approaches include the following features:

Setting a quit date: The usual recommendation is to set a quit date about two weeks hence—long enough to allow time for preparation and reflection, but not so long that it fades into the distant future. Ideally, it will be a time when you don't typically smoke a lot or are not under a high level of stress. Early April, for example, is not a great quit date for a tax preparation specialist!

Enlisting social support: If you are working with a counselor, s/he will be your best source of support because that support is focused on your particular smoking and quitting behavior. For a less-formal program, you may be encouraged to draft your spouse, friends, or coworkers to provide encouragement (and equally important, to avoid sabotaging your efforts).

Problem solving and skill building: Most programs help you to anticipate some of the challenges you'll face and offer suggestions and tips for dealing with them—how to refuse convincingly when someone offers you a cigarette, how to avoid negative self-talk ("Just this one won't hurt") and emphasize positive self-talk ("I did a good job resolving that pesky billing issue without my usual cigarette"), and how to prepare for temptations you're likely to encounter (e.g., during social occasions or when things go wrong).

Maintaining abstinence and dealing with slips: You should be very proud when you've succeeded in quitting, but don't get cocky! Temptation can strike when you least expect it, even after many months of abstinence, so once you've completed your quit program, you'll need to keep the skills you've acquired polished and ready for use.

If you slip and have a cigarette, or even several, you're likely to feel frustrated and discouraged. Remember our discussion of the abstinence violation effect in Chapter 3? It applies to smoking as well as eating. Resist the temptation to give in and say, "Oh, the heck with it." Remind yourself that a slip is just a slip, nothing more, and shouldn't be confused with a full-blown relapse. Keep your perspective: Your task is simply *not to smoke the next cigarette*. Focus on this, and everything else will fall into place.

If somehow you fall off the wagon and return to smoking, take a few deep breaths and revisit your assessment of what will work for you. You now know something about yourself that you might not have known before, and you may conclude that a more intensive intervention is needed. This has happened to many successful former smokers and should not be a cause for despair.

Finding a Formal Treatment Program
There are many good ways to find a reputable treatment program.

Ask Your Doctor

Although many health-care providers fail to do so, the current accepted standard of care specifies that all health-care encounters should include a query about smoking, a recommendation that you quit, assistance in arranging for help in doing so, and follow-up care to determine whether you succeeded. The next time you go to your doctor's office for a routine visit or nonemergency medical care, be sure to raise this topic yourself if your doctor or a staff member does not.

If you don't have an appointment coming up, give your health-care provider a call. Many health maintenance organizations (HMOs) offer their own programs or will refer you to programs for which they will reimburse you.

Organizations with Smoking-Cessation Programs

The following organizations should be able to direct you to reputable programs or clinicians in your local area:

American Cancer Society (800) ACS-2345;
http://www.cancer.org

American Heart Association (800) 242-1793

American Lung Association (800) 586-4872 or
(212) 315-8700; http://www.lungusa.org

National Cancer Institute—Cancer Information Service
(800) 4-CANCER or (800) 422-6237;
http://www.cancer.gov

Nicotine Anonymous (the twelve-step approach)
(877) TRY-NICA (877-879-6422);
http://www.nicotine-anonymous.org

Workplace Interventions

Especially if you work for a large organization, you may find your employer has discovered the cost-effectiveness of offering a smoking-cessation intervention as a health benefit.

Clinical Trials

University-based researchers, university hospitals, and large HMOs (such as Kaiser Permanente) often carry out clinical trials of new medications or new behavioral methods for quitting. This is a good way to obtain state-of-the-art treatment at little or no cost. You may, however, be assigned to a control group. Be sure to ask whether the control group receives "usual care" (that is, a currently approved method or drug) or no treatment/placebo treatment. If it is the latter, ask whether the trial includes a plan for subsequent treatment. Be aware, too, that research studies often have strict criteria regarding who can be admitted to the trial, so don't be too surprised or disappointed if you turn out to be ineligible for reasons that seem arbitrary or because you don't fall into certain categories that relate to the hypotheses being tested.

If you live near a university, particularly a large one or one with a medical school, call for information about this option, and be sure to check the classified ads in your local newspaper. And even if they aren't running any clinical trials, colleges and universities often offer other low-cost options for smoking-cessation treatment. For a listing of government-sponsored clinical trials around the country, visit: http://clinicaltrials.gov/ct/search?term=smoking+cessation.

Telephone Quitlines

Several studies have shown that telephone counseling can improve a smoker's chance of quitting successfully. In one American Cancer Society study conducted in 2000, access to counseling nearly doubled the rate of quitting maintained for at least one year.

Quitlines have received good federal support and all fifty states have now established telephone hotlines for quitting. To find a telephone quitline in your state, call (800) QUIT-NOW

(784-8669). You can also reach smoking-cessation counselors who can answer smoking-related questions in English or Spanish at the National Cancer Institute by calling (877) 44U-QUIT (448-7848).

In addition, many states have implemented "FAX-to-quit" programs that enable your health-care professional to refer you to a quitline. The quitline will then initiate a call to you, in whatever language you speak, and make arrangements for further counseling.

Web-Assisted Tobacco Interventions (WATI)

Internet-based smoking-cessation programs have proliferated, ranging from the reputable to the absurd. A significant advantage of the Internet approach is the 24/7 access it affords. The following list includes well-respected programs that have been developed by experts—though controlled trials assessing outcome remain to be conducted. These sites vary in their approaches: Some emphasize motivating and preparing the smoker for the eventual quit day, while others rely more on providing educational materials or support from counselors and peers. If you think an Internet-based program is for you, do a little "comparison shopping" to determine which one is most likely to hold your attention and maintain your motivation. Here are some good options:

* One of the most extensively used and highly regarded online cessation programs, known for its accuracy and use of interactivity, is QuitNet: http://www.quitnet.com. It includes a Spanish version as well.

* Freedom From Smoking (start at http://www.lungusa.org; click on Quit Smoking, and then click FFS) is a free online smoking-cessation clinic offered by the American Lung Association.

* Visit http://www.smokefree.gov to see your tax dollars at work. This government-sponsored site features an online smoking cessation program plus lots of other useful information designed to help you quit and stay quit.

* The Massachusetts Department of Public Health maintains a useful website: http://www.trytostop.org.

* Another excellent state website is the Arizona Smokers Helpline: http://www.ashline.org.

Self-Help Books

Dozens, and possibly hundreds, of self-help books on how to stop smoking have been written and published—often by self-styled experts or enthusiasts who want to share a method that worked for them, but many are of questionable value. The following books by recognized experts focus on postcessation weight gain and other issues important to women:

* *The How to Quit Smoking and Not Gain Weight Cookbook*, by Mary Donkersloot and Linda Hyder Ferry (Three Rivers Press, 1999).

* *How Women Can Finally Stop Smoking*, by Robert C. Klesges and Margaret DeBon (Hunter House Publishers, 1994).

* *How to Quit Smoking Without Gaining Weight*, by Bess H. Marcus, Jeffrey S. Hampl, and Edwin B. Fisher (American Lung Association, 2004).

PHARMACOLOGICAL TREATMENT OPTIONS

Regardless of the behavioral method you adopt, or even if you just decide to go cold turkey, a big decision you'll have to make is whether to use medications and, if so, which is best for you.

As of this writing, there are seven FDA-approved first-line medications. Three nicotine replacement products (gum, patch, and lozenge) are available over the counter (that is, no prescription is required). Two more—nasal spray and inhaler—are obtainable only by prescription. Two non-nicotine smoking-cessation medications, Zyban and Chantix, are also available by prescription only. (See Table 7.1 on the next page.)

All of these products roughly double your chances of long-term success in quitting and work even better when coupled with a behavioral intervention. By controlling the physiological components of addiction, they can buy you the time you need to develop strategies for dealing with the behavioral components.

As we saw in Chapter 5, "Gaining a Little and Getting Okay with It," all the nicotine replacement products and Zyban lessen weight gain while you take them, which can help to start you off on the right foot. Once you succeed in quitting, Chantix may help in controlling weight during the maintenance phase, but overall, it may not be the drug of choice if weight management during your quit attempt is an important goal.

Some people are put off by the idea of fighting nicotine with more nicotine. Be aware that, except in regard to developing fetuses, nicotine itself is not much more dangerous than caffeine. To be sure, it is highly addictive, especially when delivered quickly to the brain after being inhaled into the lungs—which, as we've seen, is how it seduces you into exposing yourself to the many other more harmful chemicals in tobacco smoke. But it is far easier to wean yourself from nicotine replacement products than from cigarettes, so look on it as a stepped approach to getting off nicotine.

There is little difference in the effectiveness of these products when they are used correctly and in adequate doses. The patch is the easiest method to use and the least obtrusive; you put it on in the morning, and nothing else is needed, nor will anyone know you're wearing it unless you tell them. Nicotine

Table 7.1: Summary of FDA-Approved First-Line Medications

NICOTINE REPLACEMENT MEDICATIONS

Nicotine patch

AVAILABILITY: Over-the-counter or by prescription

HOW TO USE: Upon awakening, apply to skin as you would a Band-Aid to a relatively hairless location (e.g., neck or waist), rotating site to minimize skin irritation. Each 24-hour patch should be removed when the next one is applied (or at bedtime if sleep disturbances occur). If you use a 16-hour patch, it should be removed at bedtime. Patches come in several doses, depending on brand. Some are intended to be used in a step-down regimen (e.g., 4 weeks using a 21 mg patch, then 2 weeks using a 14 mg patch, then 2 weeks using a 7 mg patch). Others are formulated for use at a single dose (e.g., 22 mg for heavier smokers and 11 mg for lighter smokers). Follow the directions on the package insert or consult your doctor.

HOW LONG TO USE: 8 weeks

COMMON SIDE EFFECTS: Skin irritation (apply 1% hydrocortisone cream or 0.5% triamcinolone cream to relieve), insomnia, vivid dreams

COST: Around $4/day

Nicotine gum

AVAILABILITY: Over-the-counter only

HOW TO USE: Nicotine gum (regular and flavored) comes in 2 doses (pieces): 2 mg (recommended for individuals smoking 24 or fewer cigarettes/day) and 4 mg (recommended for individuals who smoke 25 or more cigarettes/day). Chew every 1–2 hours (at least 10 pieces/-day) for the first 6 weeks, then as needed (but no more than 24 pieces/day) for an additional 6 weeks. Chewing technique is important: Chew only until a "peppery" or "flavored" taste emerges, then "park" between cheek and gum. Alternate chewing and parking for about half an hour, until taste dissipates. Avoid eating or drinking anything except water for 15 minutes prior to and during chewing.

HOW LONG TO USE: 1–3 months

COMMON SIDE EFFECTS: Mouth soreness, jaw ache, hiccups; dyspepsia (especially if nicotine is swallowed due to incorrect chewing

Table 7.1: Summary of FDA-Approved First-Line Medications (cont'd.)

technique). If gum sticks to dental work, discontinue use and consult your dentist

COST: Around $4.50/day during the first six weeks of use

Nicotine lozenge

AVAILABILITY: Over-the-counter only

HOW TO USE: The nicotine lozenge is a hard candy that comes in doses of 2 mg (recommended for smokers who smoke their first cigarette of the day more than 30 minutes after waking) or 4 mg (recommended for smokers who smoke their first cigarette of the day within 30 minutes of waking). Allow the lozenge to dissolve in the mouth rather than chewing or swallowing it. Each lozenge will last about 20–30 minutes and nicotine will continue to leach through the lining of the mouth for a short time after the lozenge has disappeared. During the first 6 weeks, use 1 lozenge every 1–2 hours (minimum of 9 lozenges); in weeks 7–9, reduce use to every 24 hours; weeks 10–12, use every 4–8 hours. Do not exceed 20 lozenges per day. Avoid eating or drinking anything except water for 15 minutes prior to and during use.

HOW LONG TO USE: Up to 12 weeks

COMMON SIDE EFFECTS: Nausea, hiccups, heartburn; headache and cough with 4 mg lozenge

COST: Around $6/day for average usage (12 doses) and up to $12/day for maximum usage (20 doses) during the first 6 weeks of use

Nicotine inhaler

AVAILABILITY: By prescription only

HOW TO USE: The plastic cylinder contains a cartridge that delivers nicotine vapor when puffed on. Use frequently in response to craving. Each cartridge delivers a total of 4 mg of nicotine over 80 inhalations, 2 of which are actually absorbed. Recommended dosage is at least 6 but not more than 16 cartridges/day. Avoid eating or drinking anything except water for 15 minutes prior to and during use. Nicotine delivery is significantly reduced at ambient temperatures of less than 50°F, so keep in an inside pocket in cold weather.

(cont'd.)

Table 7.1: Summary of FDA-Approved First-Line Medications (cont'd.)

How Long to Use: Up to 6 months, tapering use during the second 3 months

Common Side Effects: Local irritation of the throat and mouth; coughing. Both should decline with continued use

Cost: Around $7–$19/day, depending on amount used

Nicotine nasal spray

Availability: By prescription only

How to Use: Nicotine nasal spray is dispensed from a pump bottle similar to over-the-counter decongestant sprays. A single dose is two sprays of 0.5 mg each, one in each nostril, for a total of 1 mg. To administer, tilt the head back slightly, and insert the tip of the bottle as far as is comfortable into the nostril. Breathe through the mouth while spraying, being careful not to sniff or inhale. Each bottle contains around 100 doses. The minimum recommended dose is 8 doses/day and the maximum is 40 doses/day (5 doses per hour).

How Long to Use: 3–6 months

Common Side Effects: Nose and throat irritation; nasal congestion; transient changes in taste, smell

Cost: Around $4–$20/day, depending on amount used

NON-NICOTINE MEDICATIONS

Zyban (bupropion SR)

Availability: By prescription only

How to Use: Treatment (orally administered tablets) should begin one week prior to the quit date. For the first 3 days, take 150 mg/day every morning; starting on Day 4, take 150 mg twice daily, with at least 8 hours between doses, for a total of 300 mg/day. Use alcohol only in moderation.

How Long to Use: 7–12 weeks; can be used for up to 6 months at 150 mg/day postquit; discontinue if there is no significant progress by Week 7

Common Side Effects: Insomnia, dry mouth; rarely, serious psychiatric side effects

Cost: Around $7/day ($3.50/day for generic version)

Table 7.1: Summary of FDA-Approved First-Line Medications (cont'd.)

Chantix (varenicline)

AVAILABILITY: By prescription only

HOW TO USE: Treatment (orally administered tablets) should begin one week prior to the quit date. For the first 3 days, take 0.5 mg/day every morning; on days 4–7, take 0.5 mg twice daily; starting on Day 8 (quit day), take 1.0 mg twice daily. Take on a full stomach; avoid taking at bedtime to minimize insomnia.

HOW LONG TO USE: 12 weeks. Can be doubled in those who have successfully quit to maximize chances of remaining smoke free.

COMMON SIDE EFFECTS: Nausea, insomnia, vivid dreams; rarely, serious psychiatric side effects

COST: Around $4.50/day

is absorbed steadily through the skin, building up in your bloodstream in about three hours. Most patches are intended for twenty-four-hour use, but a sixteen-hour patch is also available. The latter is less likely to cause sleep disturbances and strange, vivid dreams, but you're more likely to wake up in a state of nicotine withdrawal.

The other nicotine replacement products have a feature that neither the patch nor the non-nicotine drugs can boast— namely, that they can be used acutely in response to an urge to smoke. With three of them—gum, lozenge, and inhaler—nicotine is absorbed through the buccal glands in the mouth; with the nasal spray, nicotine is absorbed through the nasal membranes. The inhaler—a cylindrical device that you puff on like a cigarette, provides the best replacement for the "handling" aspects of smoking but has the drawback of taking fifteen to twenty minutes to finish "puffing" the nicotine vapor each time you use it. The nasal spray takes effect very quickly, so it may hold a particular appeal for highly dependent smokers.

(For the same reason, it is the hardest of the smoking-cessation drugs to give up.) The gum is probably the second-most effective, after the nasal spray, in providing prompt relief of craving, but this aid depends on mastery of the "chew and park" technique to work properly. All four products have the feature of giving you something you can do (other than smoke) when you're assaulted by a craving for a cigarette. Note, however, that especially at the beginning of treatment, a fixed schedule of administration (rather than waiting for a craving to occur) is advised in some instances in order to assure adequate dosing and a buildup of nicotine concentrations in the blood.

Zyban (bupropion hydrochloride) started life as Wellbutrin, an atypical antidepressant that acts by inhibiting the reuptake of norepinephrine. It took on a new incarnation when Dr. Linda Ferry, chief of preventive medicine at the Veterans Affairs Medical Center in Loma Linda, California, started looking for a drug that might improve the dismal quit rate at the VA Medical Center's smoking-cessation clinic by stabilizing brain chemistry and reducing the need for nicotine. Prozac had been tested as a stop-smoking aid without much success, but knowing that approximately half the smokers treated in her clinic had symptoms of depression, Dr. Ferry hoped that some other antidepressant might show better results. When a colleague mentioned that depressed patients treated with Wellbutrin reported not only an improvement in mood but also less craving for coffee, chocolate, and cigarettes, Ferry decided to set up a small trial, using funds from the university to cover drugs and lab tests and recruiting her mother to serve as her research assistant. Her initial results were so promising that the manufacturer went on to conduct larger trials, and, in 1997, Zyban became the first non-nicotine smoking cessation aid to receive FDA approval.

Ironically, given its history, Zyban works as well in helping nondepressed smokers to quit as it does in depressed smokers. This is probably because, in addition to its antidepressant effects, the drug also directly prevents nicotine's actions. Nonetheless, if you are prone to depression, Zyban may be a good choice for you. Like nicotine replacement products, it also has weight-suppressing effects. Note, however, that since Zyban lowers seizure threshold, it should not be used by people with a history of seizures or eating disorders (a risk factor for seizures—possibly because of dehydration or the effects of long-term malnutrition on the brain).

The other FDA-approved non-nicotine smoking-cessation aid is Chantix (varenicline tartrate; sold as Champix in Europe). Unlike Zyban, Chantix was specifically designed to treat nicotine addiction, based on its effects on nicotinic receptors in the brain. It works in two ways—by reducing the pleasure of smoking and by alleviating withdrawal symptoms. It does this very well and has perhaps the best success rate of all approved drugs, even in highly dependent smokers. At least one study has shown positive effects on mood and cognition during smoking abstinence. As noted in Chapter 5, it has little impact on weight.

Some of the initial enthusiasm for Zyban and Chantix has been tempered by occasional reports of serious psychiatric side effects. On July 1, 2009, after reviewing these concerns, the FDA announced that it would require the manufacturers of these drugs to include a warning label highlighting the risk of changes in behavior, depressed mood, hostility, and suicidal thoughts. Janet Woodcock, MD, director of the FDA's Center for Drug Evaluation and Research, stated in the press release that "Smoking is the leading cause of preventable disease, disability, and death in the United States and we know these products are effective aids in helping people quit." The document further noted that neither Zyban nor Chantix contains nicotine, and some of the observed symptoms may be a response to nicotine withdrawal rather than a direct effect of the drugs themselves. The fact that the formulations and mode of action of the two drugs are quite different lends support to this conjecture. Nonetheless, until controlled trials have established or ruled out a causal connection, these medications must be used with caution. Please make sure your health-care professional is aware of your medical history before reaching a decision about prescribing either of these drugs. If after consultation you decide to try one, keep in close touch with her/-him and report any changes in mood or behavior you notice.

Since all the FDA-approved drugs address different aspects of nicotine dependence, it makes sense to ask if they can be combined. Yes, in fact, they can. Combinations of first-line medications that can further improve chances of successful quitting include patch combined with gum, patch combined with nasal spray, patch combined with inhaler, and patch combined with Zyban. Additional combinations will likely be tested in the future.

Not everyone should use these medications. There is no good evidence to support the use of medications in light or nondaily smokers—and at least for nicotine replacement products, you may actually expose your body to nicotine in doses that may be excessive or even toxic for you. Pregnant women should exhaust all other options for quitting before using any pharmacotherapy (remembering, however, that they are exposing their unborn child to a jolt of nicotine each time they light up); the same is true for nursing mothers. Adolescents and people with serious medical conditions should seek medical advice before using any of these products.

A number of other drugs have shown some promise as aids to smoking cessation, including clonidine (an antihypertensive that has also been tested for a variety of other conditions including alcohol and narcotic withdrawal) and nortriptiline (an antidepressant). These are available only by prescription and can be discussed with your physician if the first-line medications do not work or are contraindicated. There are also many herbal products available claiming to promote quitting, but *none of these has been approved by the FDA.*

Also warranting mention are attempts to create less harmful tobacco products (e.g., preparations that use genetically modified or detoxified tobacco, preparations intended to be chewed rather than smoked, etc.), and alternative nicotine delivery devices (most notably the electronic cigarette, also known as the e-cigarette, a battery-powered device delivering a vaporized propylene glycol/nicotine solution via inhalation). These products are not manufactured by the pharmaceutical industry and are not explicitly marketed as smoking-cessation devices. Rather, they are intended to provide safe or safer alternatives for delivering nicotine—in other words, to create or maintain nicotine addiction with fewer or none of the hazards of inhaled tobacco smoke. Many, if not all, of these products are undoubtedly safer than the cigarette. (Indeed, it would be difficult to devise something *more* lethal!) The question is whether they are *enough* safer to justify risking primary addiction by children and adolescents and relinquishing the hope of persuading addicted smokers to give up nicotine altogether. It seems unlikely that combustible products will meet that test, but some of the other formulations show promise for the future, pending further research. Again, *none of these has been approved by the FDA.*

THE ECONOMICS OF QUITTING

The Institute of Medicine has recommended that all insurance, managed-care, and employee benefit plans, including Medicaid, cover reimbursement for effective smoking-cessation programs. Unfortunately, we aren't there yet, and patterns of coverage in this country are a bit of a patchwork quilt. Why should this be? I think it may just one more manifestation of our lingering ambivalence about this problem, fed by the tobacco industry's continued insistence that smoking is a "pleasant adult custom" that the smoker could give up if she chose. I still remember my surprise the first time I heard the term "lifestyle drug," a category in which smoking-cessation medications are lumped together with hair loss and erectile dysfunction preparations. Add to this the widespread suspicion of the motives of so-called "Big Pharma" and the feeling that the Tobacco Settlement funds were supposed to be used for this purpose (though in many states they were not), and no wonder it is so hard to persuade politicians to vote to mandate this benefit.

For most smokers, however, there are some, if not many, options available—though you may need to do some digging to identify them. For starters, many of the programs listed above are low-cost or free. (If you enroll in a clinical trial, you may even receive a modest compensation for participating.)

If you decide to seek professional counseling and/or medication, find out what is covered by your insurance. If you are a state employee, you may be in luck: More than half of all states cover at least one Public Health Service-recommended treatment, although only a handful offer the full spectrum.

Around 75 percent of state Medicaid programs offer at least one form of tobacco dependence treatment, including one or more forms of medication. A handful offer coverage only for pregnant women. New states periodically join those states covering smoking-cessation treatment or expand existing coverage, but at least three states have actually scaled back coverage.

For individuals with smoking-related diseases, Medicare will cover two cessation attempts per year. Each attempt may include a maximum of four intermediate (three to ten minutes) or intensive (more than ten minutes) counseling sessions, with the total annual benefit covering up to eight sessions in a twelve-month period. In addition, Medicare Part D will cover medications prescribed by a physician, though it will not cover over-the-counter treatments.

When you think about the money it costs to quit, don't forget to balance it against the money it costs to smoke. If you're a pack-a-day smoker, not buying cigarettes gives you close to a $2,000 subsidy toward whatever quit program you choose!

A FINAL WORD OF CAUTION

A deep-seated ambivalence persists among the people who do research on smoking about the importance of weight gain as a barrier to quitting. Reasons for this ambivalence have been discussed throughout this book. They have to do with conflicting results of clinical trials that include weight control components, failure to take into account the many women who never even try to quit because of the fear of gaining weight, a desire to meet the needs of all smokers whether or not they are weight concerned, and, in some quarters, difficulty in understanding that concerns about weight and appearance have to be addressed in their own right, not as being in a seesaw relationship with concerns about health. So please use the information and advice provided in this book to help you choose a smoking-cessation method that treats concerns about weight and physical appearance with dignity, and to supplement your method of choice as needed.

8

The Chic of Quitting

According to the medical dictionary on my bookshelf, *health* is "a state of optimal physical, mental, and social well-being." Good health isn't simply the absence of disease or infirmity; it is something that radiates from the core of your being. Health and beauty are natural allies. When they are in conflict, something has gone awry.

Good health is something we often don't think about until we don't have it. Of course, no one can be 100 percent healthy 100 percent of the time. Our genetics, our history, our environment—all these factors play a role in shaping our potential for physical and psychological health. There is grace and wisdom in accepting what can't be changed and playing out the hand we've been dealt. But many things *are* under our control or can be brought under our control, and we can take steps to ensure that we've come as close as we can to fulfilling our personal potential for good health.

That's not to say that we don't all take risks with our health. Every time we get into a car or cross a street, we take a small but measurable risk with our health. We're all willing to accept some degree of risk in order to achieve certain benefits; otherwise, what's the point of living? Everyone has her own sense of what constitutes an acceptable risk. The same person who says he can't understand why a woman would take risks with her health in order to be slim may drive at breakneck speeds to get to the ski slopes for the weekend—as though the thrill of hurtling down a mountain on slats of high-tech plastic at forty-five miles per hour is somehow a higher order of benefit than the confidence and contentment that comes with looking your best—*fare bella figura*.

The problem with cigarette smoking is not just that it is a health risk, but that it is a bad bargain—definitely over the long run, and often over the not-so-long run. *You don't get what you pay for, you pay too much for what you do get, and you can find better ways to get the results you want.* At best, smoking substitutes the appearance of health for health itself. A woman in a treatment group quoted by Klesges and DeBon in *How Women Can Finally Stop Smoking*, when reminded of the tradeoff she was making in smoking to achieve slimness, wryly quipped, "But think how great I'll look in my coffin!" Sadly, bad health outcomes tend to seep like an oil spill into all aspects of life; all too often, they defeat the hope that smoking will improve physical appearance not only in the coffin but also during one's stay on this planet.

This point was recently brought home to me with great poignance. While vacationing in New Mexico, my husband and I went for a hike in the Bandelier National Monument, a stunning, unforgiving landscape of red clay escarpments, dotted with ancient Pueblo cave dwellings accessible only by ladder. As I sat in the parking lot waiting for my husband to emerge from the Visitors' Center, an elderly couple trudged slowly past me. The man was sprightly and trim, with an astonishing shock of pure white hair. The woman, perfectly coiffed and dressed in an attractive lime-green shell with pink-and-green plaid shorts, leaned heavily on his arm. That she had once been beautiful was clear, but the ravages of disease had taken their toll. Alas, "slender" would be a generous description of her haggard, wasted frame. Her slow pace was explained by the oxygen tank her husband wheeled along with his other hand.

I admired her grit and his devotion, but mainly I was awash with pity at their plight—and with anger at the tobacco industry for luring them into it. For although I didn't have access to her medical history, it is a pretty safe bet that the woman was a long-term smoker and was now paying a high price in the form of chronic obstructive pulmonary disease (COPD), the collective term for chronic bronchitis and emphysema. About 90 percent of COPD deaths are caused by smoking. Despite the obvious pains she took with her appearance, there is nothing attractive about end-stage COPD. In some ways, COPD can be a worse scourge than lung cancer because the disease can linger for years, during which the victim gulps painfully for air without ever getting quite enough oxygen. It is slow death by drowning—air, air everywhere, and not a drop to breathe. And to use the cliché that someone always trots out when hard lessons are learned too late, it didn't have to happen.

When you become a nonsmoker, you take a giant step toward assuring that it won't happen to you.

FIRST THE BAD NEWS...

So far I haven't spoken much about the health effects of smoking. It is hard to scare people into stopping, because they tend to tune out messages they don't want to hear. In this "go for the gusto" society of ours, people persuade themselves that smoking is "going for the gusto." "Life is more than longevity," they intone, or "Smoking is cool," or "You could get hit by a bus tomorrow." Psychologists have a term for arguments like these: *postdecisional dissonance*. Basically, it means that once you've decided to do something, or gotten hooked on doing something, you'll be much more receptive to ideas that are consistent with or reinforce that decision than to ideas that challenge or devalue it.

To appreciate fully the changes that come with quitting, however, you need at least a little background on what smoking does to a woman's body in the first place. And now that you're a nonsmoker or on the verge of becoming one, you should be able to put these facts into perspective.

If you were to ask the man or woman on the street to identify the leading cause of cancer deaths in women, odds are that the majority would guess breast cancer. In fact, at some point in the mid-1980s, lung cancer surpassed breast cancer as the leading cause of cancer death in women. Let me repeat that: *Lung cancer kills more women than breast cancer*—nearly twice as many, an estimated seventy-three thousand in 2005, compared with forty thousand breast cancer victims. A little of this positional change is accounted for by improvements in breast cancer survival, but most of it is due to increases in lung cancer. Lung cancer deaths among women have increased by 600 percent since 1950—a ripple effect from the uptake of smoking among women a few decades ago. Indeed, the change is almost entirely accounted for by smoking; the rate of lung cancer among nonsmokers has remained low and stable.

It is hardly surprising that breast cancer springs to mind when the subject of cancer in women comes up. Advocates for breast cancer research have been very effective in lobbying for their cause. They solicit sponsors for women on three-day breast cancer walks and "wear-denim-to-work" days; they distribute pink ribbons to bring attention to the issue. Proceeds from a breast cancer postage stamp go to support breast cancer research.

Lung cancer, by contrast, is the elephant in the living room. Not for a moment do I begrudge the advocates for breast cancer research their success in their efforts to combat a disease that so tragically affects the lives of many women and those who love them, but I often ask myself why lung cancer is virtually invisible by comparison. I suspect the answer, at least in part, is that breast cancer seems to strike randomly; no woman can feel completely confident that she will not be the next to fall victim to this disease. Lung cancer, on the other hand, is largely confined to people who engage in a behavior that many regard as voluntary, so the element of "blame the victim" starts to creep in. In fact, smokers may actually blame themselves. Women are especially good at that!

If you've stayed with me this far, you know better by now. You know that women are seduced into smoking when they are too young to make an informed choice, only to discover later that they've been hooked on an addictive substance that suppresses body weight and helps in mood management, delivered in a very dangerous package. You know that, just as some women are genetically at greatly increased risk of breast cancer, some are also genetically at greatly increased risk of smoking. You know that whenever one woman falls prey to a smoking-related disease, all women are diminished.

Lung cancer, while the most common of smoking-related cancers, isn't the only one. Smoking is also a risk factor for cancers of the cervix, mouth, larynx (voice box), esophagus, pharynx (throat), kidney, bladder, pancreas, liver, stomach, colon, and rectum, as well as some forms of leukemia.

But by far the biggest smoking-related killer of women isn't cancer at all: It is heart disease. Regardless of smoking status, heart disease kills more women than all forms of cancer combined. Yet according to the American Heart Association, 43 percent of women are unaware that heart disease is the number one cause of death among women. Many still think of heart disease as a "man's disease"—a dangerous myth. That's probably because women tend to develop heart disease later than men, with most deaths occurring after menopause. Smoking undercuts some of this protection, however, increasing the risk more in younger women than in older women. Women who smoke are also at greatly increased risk of stroke. Smoking, in combination with taking birth control pills, disastrously multiplies the risk of heart disease and stroke, especially in women over the age of thirty-five.

Smoking can seriously undermine the health of your reproductive system. As we saw in Chapter 1, smokers enter menopause a year or two earlier, on average, than women who have never smoked, and they have a higher risk of infertility. Smoking is associated with higher rates of cervical dysplasia, a precancerous condition that can be diagnosed by Pap smear, and subsequent progression to cervical cancer. Women who smoke during pregnancy have a higher risk of the placenta growing too close to the opening of the uterus, premature membrane rupture, and placentas that separate from the uterus too early, which can lead to bleeding, premature delivery, and emergency Caesarean section.

Smoking can also affect your children's health. Smoking during pregnancy is linked to low birth weight and a two- to threefold risk of sudden infant death syndrome, or SIDS. Exposure to secondhand smoke in the home increases the risk of asthma, pneumonia, bronchitis, and fluid in the middle ear. And if you smoke, your children are more likely to smoke, too.

...AND NOW THE GOOD NEWS

What happens to your body when you quit smoking? The good news is that some smoking-related changes will regress so that it will be almost as though you had never smoked at all. Others may not regress fully, or at all, but, even so, stopping smoking will halt further progression.

Predictably, much of the research on the nature of and timetable for the effects of quitting has focused on the major health benefits—reductions in the risk of heart disease, cancer, and lung disease. To summarize briefly, quitting smoking decreases the risk of all of the above in comparison with continued smoking. The risk of cardiovascular disease drops to half that of a smoker by one year, reverting completely by fifteen years. Stroke risk decreases in a similar timeframe. Lung cancer risk, though tapering off more slowly and less completely reversible than that of heart disease, declines to about half that of a smoker in ten years. Some improvements occur quite rapidly; for example, clotting ability, which is impaired by smoking, returns to normal within two weeks. The younger you are when you quit, the greater the risk reduction. The risk of death from all causes among former smokers approaches the level of never-smokers ten to fourteen years after cessation. It is never too late to quit; stopping at age sixty-five or older reduces risk of dying from a smoking-related disease by nearly one-half.

You also reduce your risk of cervical dysplasia when you stop smoking. If you already have cervical dysplasia, quitting smoking reduces your risk of progression to cervical cancer. Unlike many smoking-related cancers, cervical cancer can and often does strike relatively early in life, and quitting can actually reverse precancerous changes rather rapidly. This is one of the best "good news" stories about quitting smoking that I know of. Any young woman who cares about preserving her reproductive options will throw away her cigarettes as fast as she can.

Considerable research has been devoted to the implications of quitting smoking for the developing fetus. If you quit smoking before pregnancy or within the first three to four months, your risk of having a low birth-weight baby becomes comparable to that of a never-smoking mom. Avoiding exposing your unborn child to nicotine and the other constituents of smoked tobacco substantially reduces risk of ectopic pregnancy, placental problems, premature rupture of membranes, miscarriage, preterm delivery, and stillbirth. Babies born to nonsmoking mothers have half the risk of sudden infant death syndrome. Sparing infants and children exposure to environmental tobacco smoke decreases the severity of asthma and other respiratory diseases. For women who have children or are planning to have them, this is a huge benefit of quitting.

These changes are all to the good, but you're also interested in how quitting affects how you look and feel; otherwise, you wouldn't be reading this book. The removal of the weight-suppressing effects of nicotine is bothersome for most quitters and may be a particular challenge for someone like you. But with this book in your hands, you're ready to deal with that challenge. Reread this book, especially the sections that apply to you; check out my recommendations for further reading at the end of the book.

Less is known about the effects of quitting on other aspects of appearance, such as skin, hair, nails, and teeth. Obviously, some of the "mechanical" effects of smoking—discolorations of skin and nails, burns on your clothes, etc.—go away completely when smoking ceases. Your breath and your clothes will smell cleaner and fresher—not to mention your furniture and your car. Regarding other effects, an important and encouraging clue is that age of menopause in former smokers is comparable to that of women who have never smoked—suggesting that the aging effects of smoking are not only halted but at least to some extent reversible. Women with concerns related to appearance and body image can also take heart from the following findings:

* Former smokers run a lower risk of gum disease than current smokers. Risk of tooth loss in former smokers is also decreased.

* Former smokers show greater bone mass than current smokers, suggesting that smoking cessation halts or slows bone loss and osteoporosis.

* Risk of cataracts in former smokers is reduced from that of current smokers.

Something I once wanted to do was to create a website to which a woman smoker could submit a current photograph. The big idea was to use age-progression techniques—what the police use to visualize how someone who has been missing for several years might look today—to project two different options: (1) how she would look ten years or twenty years from now if she continued to smoke; and (2) how she would look in ten or twenty years if she quit smoking today. The result would be something like the identical twin photos that I mentioned in Chapter 1—except that the images would be of the smoker herself, not of some stranger. The keep-on-smoking version would have more wrinkles, grayer hair, and other signs of more rapid aging than the stop-smoking version. The smoker would probably be slightly thinner but also—the flip side of thinner—more haggard and less shapely.

Even though I never had the chance to carry out this project, you can do it as a thought experiment—or even try modifying a photo of yourself with a pen or a computer. Using this method—no cheating!—it shouldn't be too hard to convince yourself that the future you will be a more attractive woman if you quit smoking, as long as you avoid excessive weight gain (which is what this book is all about).

BEYOND *CARPE DIEM*

Why is it so easy to understand what's wrong with smoking, overeating, and underexercising, and yet so hard to modify these behaviors? If we were Vulcans, like Mr. Spock, governed purely by logic, we'd all do the right thing. For us Earthlings, however, immediate and reliable rewards, even if they are small, can outweigh longer-term or iffier benefits, even if they are large. That chocolate truffle or that cigarette sitting right in front of us exerts a stronger influence than the promise of good health at some unspecified future time. The "benefits" of not exercising—more time for other activities, less risk of injury, less expense for special clothes and equipment, and avoiding feelings of self-consciousness or intimidation—make exercising easier to duck, despite the well-known positive effects of physical activity on health, fitness, and appearance. And it is not all psychological. A bite of chocolate or a puff of tobacco smoke can cause changes in our "internal milieu" that give us a brief psychological lift; not exercising lets us avoid the feeling of fatigue or muscle soreness that follows exercise.

Undoubtedly, being responsive to immediate rewards conferred some advantage at one time in human history. Before advances in modern medicine enabled large numbers of us to live into old age, many died of infectious disease, lack of food, or loss of teeth long before the consequences of poor nutrition or a sedentary lifestyle had a chance to take their toll. Moreover, during large portions of human history, having too little food and leisure were greater problems for our ancestors than having too much. *Carpe diem* was the key to survival.

Well, in an age of plenty, *carpe diem*—"seize the day," or, more colloquially, grab opportunity when it strikes—is fine for special occasions (eating a slice of wedding cake or skipping your workout when your sister flies in for a visit). But if you "seize the day" every day and turn it into a way of life—spending most of October eating the candy you bought to distribute to trick-or-treaters, or ducking out of your workout day after day just to snatch a few extra zzz's—you lose the sense of specialness. More importantly, you lose the sense that you're in charge of your own body—what you put into it and what you do with it.

Acute attacks of "willpower" aren't likely to work for most people. Good intentions, embraced in a burst of enthusiasm, tend not to survive moments when you're tired or rushed or feeling blue. My aerobics class always swells at the beginning of January with people whose New Year's resolution to exercise generally evaporates by the end of the month. What I've tried to suggest in this book are ways to restructure your environment and restructure your thinking so that it is easy and fun to do the right thing. As you master these techniques, it should become easier, not harder, because the results of your efforts provide their own rewards, and because you've learned not to let occasional slips drag you back into self-defeating patterns.

THE CHIC OF QUITTING

Of course, you cannot go back and become a person who has never smoked. Regrets may be useful if they help you and others learn from past mistakes and avoid making bad decisions in the future. Dwelling excessively on the past, however, is not conducive to happiness. It should be relatively easy to forgive yourself for starting and continuing to smoke when you consider the massive efforts of an enormous industry to seduce people before they have reached the age of consent into using an addictive product. The important thing now is to move forward and deal with what you can exert some control over—the future.

Over the years, my work has brought me into contact with many people who have quit smoking. Some of them never get beyond the point of having simply subtracted tobacco from their lives. They have *given up* smoking. They know they've sacrificed their cigarettes in the service of better health, and they're glad not to have their spouse and children nagging at them to quit. Eventually, as the craving subsides and the environmental cues associated with smoking break down, they may pretty much forget about smoking, or they may go on missing their cigarettes but pushing it out of their minds.

That's okay—whatever works. There are some nonsmokers, however, who seem to find a way to make the process more creative, to walk away from cigarettes with something positive. They are to be envied. Earlier in this book I spoke of mindful eating, mindful drinking, mindful exercising. Let's talk about yet another form of mindfulness, one that's only open to former smokers, and that is *mindful nonsmoking*. On a website developed by a former smoker named Terry Martin, I found the reflections of several women (including Terry herself) who have used the process of quitting as a springboard to achieving higher levels of comfort, confidence, and awareness:

> "I have found a peace that I never experienced before… an awareness of my world and everything in it. I have an abundance of energy, a joy in living, more confidence than ever before."
>
> — Anna (http://quitsmoking.about.com/ cs/ourstories/a/annaquitstory.htm)

> "I have discovered a new life since I quit smoking. My health has greatly improved, my house smells fresh, and so do I. When my grandson comes over, I spend precious time with him instead of wondering how I am going to

sneak outside for a puff. My husband and I have learned how to have a conversation with each other again instead of sitting and smoking our quality time away. We both go for long walks and enjoy each other's company as it should be…. I always look at my quitting smoking as a gift I am giving to myself. The gift of life—how [much] more precious can this be! I was a smoker for 33 years, and for the first time in my life, I feel freedom is mine, and I cherish it with each passing moment."

— Jan (http://quitsmoking.about.com/od/
quitsmokingstories/a/JanQuitStory.htm)

"I've gotten into the habit of using gratitude on a daily basis. This new life I've created for myself is a precious gift that I cherish and nurture. I love my life so much more now that I'm not living it in a cloud of smoke. It's been said that gratitude unlocks the fullness of life, and I believe that. I used it as a tool to help remind me of my progress, and it has rewarded me with an increased awareness for all of the many blessings elsewhere in my life. The cigarette-induced anxiety I suffered is gone, I'm delighted to say. Life is good."

— Terry (http://quitsmoking.about.com/
cs/ourstories/a/mystory.htm)

"I know that some people do gain a little weight after they quit, but I'm here to tell you that NOT EVERYONE WILL GAIN WEIGHT. Don't let that fear stand in the way of the best decision you will ever make in your life. I truly believe that I would never have lost weight if I was still smoking. I've used the extra energy that I've got from cessation to become more active and more involved in life. I don't want to be on the sidelines anymore. Quitting smoking will create such amazing change in the rest of your life. It is not always an easy path, but it is SO worth it. I celebrated my 6-month milestone yesterday, and I can promise that I will NEVER go back to smoking. I have gained so much [in my life], and I absolutely refuse to let it go. I'm truly happy for the first time in years. I look forward to the future, and I get excited about new challenges. I feel awesome, and I LOVE my life."

— Maia (http://quitsmoking.about.com/cs/sixmomilestones/a/msmojo6months.htm)

"I believe we have used smoking for so much emotional repression, that food just sort of takes the place of the fumes in filling the void. I also still maintain that [it is] better to carry a few pounds around that can eventually be lost, than an oxygen tank! And so what about a few pounds!…My skin is absolutely glowing! My eyes are bright, my breath is fresh, and I've gotten some double takes when I've been out and about. There's nothing sexier than health and confidence, and quitting smoking gives you both. In spades."

— Leslie (http://quitsmoking.about.com/od/weightgain/a/thechubster.htm)

These women understand that quitting isn't just a matter of weaning oneself from cigarettes. Some of them have done what they needed to do to maintain or lose weight; others have decided to tolerate a few extra pounds. Some had to overcome depression. None of them found quitting easy. But they have all learned that the benefits of quitting go beyond the diseases that they won't get and the money that they won't waste—not that these aren't important, but they don't fully capture the joy of being a nonsmoker after having been a smoker. All of these women exemplify what I like to think of as the "chic of quitting."

As I noted at the start of our journey, this book is about personal style, about regaining control of your life, about letting go of smoking and the comforts it provides by finding other ways to feel good about yourself and to look terrific. Few things, including smoking, are so thoroughly bad that a wise person can't extract something good from them. If you have mastered the principles outlined in this book, you have learned some life skills that you might have missed had you never smoked. Now that you no longer spend your time half-listening to friends or only partly absorbed in what you're doing because you're always planning your next smoke, you can fully grasp the meaning of "living in the moment." The resulting positive attitude about your new nonsmoking self and your body is truly the chic of quitting.

Additional Reading and Resources for Weight and Mood Management

The following list of resources, organized to accompany chapters in this book, includes some of my personal favorites but should not be regarded as exhaustive. If you discover a website or book or product that you think should be included, please write or e-mail me, and I'll consider your suggestion for inclusion in subsequent editions or posting on the *Life After Cigarettes* website.

Some of the books I've recommended may be out of print, but used or remaindered copies can usually be obtained at http://www.amazon.com or http://www.half.com.

Websites can come and go in the blink of an eye, but all URLs cited below were verified shortly before publication and were correct as of summer, 2009.

Disclaimer: I have no financial interest in any of the products or services mentioned below or in any other part of this book.

Commonsense Precautions: Be a careful consumer. Before you use any information on a listed website or buy any listed product, satisfy yourself that the website is reliable and that the product will meet your needs.

Dietary Management (Chapter 3 Resources)

A graphic representation and explanation of the somewhat confusing "food pyramid" can be found at http://www.MyPyramid.gov.

If you're willing to pay for an Internet-based program, take a look at http://www.ediets.com, which offers a fair amount of flexibility and dietary choice.

Another popular and easy-to-use health and fitness program is Keyoe's "Diet and Exercise Assistant": http://www.keyoe.com. It comes in both personal digital assistant (PDA) and desktop versions.

Already mentioned is *The How to Quit Smoking and Not Gain Weight Cookbook*, by Mary Donkersloot and Linda Hyder Ferry (Three Rivers Press, 1999). Written by a nutritionist and a clinician-researcher specializing in smoking cessation, this book provides a heart-healthy diet plan, complete with recipes, as well as behavioral stop-smoking and weight management strategies.

Francophiles, check out *French Women Don't Get Fat* (Knopf, 2005), which spent many months on the best-seller list, and *French Women for All Seasons: A Year of Secrets, Recipes, and Pleasure* (Knopf, 2006). Mireille Guiliano is the author of these compilations of wise and witty observations on French women and how they manage to stay slender and look put-together without dieting or working out. (Hint: This doesn't mean they don't control their eating or engage in physical activity!) You might also wish to take a look at *Chic & Slim, Chic & Slim Encore, Armoire Boudoir Cuisine & Savvy,* and *Chic & Slim le Website* (http://www.annebarone.com) by Anne Barone, a series with a similar theme, though less recipe oriented.

Eat, Drink and Be Healthy: The Harvard Medical School Guide to Healthy Eating, by Walter C. Willett, MD, DrPH (Free Press, 2002), is an informative guide that can help you thread your way through the masses of information and misinformation about food and nutrition with which we're bombarded on a daily basis. The author is professor of Epidemiology and Nutrition and chair of the Department of Nutrition at the Harvard School of Public Health, and professor of medicine at the Harvard Medical School, Brigham and Women's Hospital. He is the principal investigator of the Nurses' Health Study II, designed to examine the association between lifestyle and nutritional factors and the occurrence of breast cancer and other major illnesses.

Exercise (Chapter 4 Resources)

Collage Video is an excellent source of exercise videos, audiotapes, and DVDs. Products are classified according to type of exercise and degree of difficulty. Many options are offered to meet special needs (e.g., pregnancy; exercises that can be done while seated; exercises appropriate for people with back pain). The fitness industry is constantly looking for ways to prevent boredom and keep people buying their products, so watch for the Hula Workout, Zumba (Latin dance adaptations), belly-dancing workouts, and other novel approaches to exercise. One-minute samples can be viewed on the Collage Video website to give you a preview of the routine and the instructor. You can also purchase accessories and equipment. Visit their website at http://www.CollageVideo.com, or call (800) 433-6769 and request a catalog. If you already know what you're looking for, Amazon.com and eBay.com are also good options.

Video-game fans looking for something a little bit different might want to look into *Dance, Dance, Revolution (DDR)*, which demos the steps to a dance and then challenges you to reproduce those steps on a mat on the floor, awarding points for successful replication. Check the following website for stand-alone, Wii, or Xbox versions: http://www.ddrgame.com.

A video/DVD series that deserves special mention is Jodi Stolove's Chair Dancing series. No more excuses about not having enough room in your small apartment; you can get a surprisingly good workout without leaving your chair! No more forgetting your towel or water bottle, or leaving your gym shoes at home. These workouts are ideal for anyone whose mobility is either temporarily or permanently restricted because of injury, infirmity, or age. The workouts are also good for any woman who does not like the feeling of moving her body around the floor or who feels self-conscious about doing so. (Many overweight women fall into this category.) In my opinion, this series is the starter exercise of choice for anyone who has no history of exercise and is not young and agile. I discovered these wonderful videos when I had a broken ankle and have returned to them frequently whenever my knee problems act up, making step aerobics uncomfortable. Each video—aerobics, toning, and yoga workouts are available—features a broad range of role models, including pregnant women, obese women, children, elderly women, and men of varying ages. They can be ordered though the Chair Dancing website, http://www.chairdancing.com, or from http://www.amazon.com.

The Anytime, Anywhere Exercise Book, by Joan Price, with Lawrence Kassman (Barnes & Noble Books, 2003), is a wonderful little book providing instructions for more than three hundred quick and easy exercises that you can do, as the title says, anytime, anywhere.

Gaiam (http://www.gaiam.com) offers online shopping for clothing, equipment, props, instructional videos, and accessories needed for yoga, Pilates, t'ai chi, and BalanceBall. These attractive, high-quality (but expensive) products are designed primarily for women.

For many women, walking is the simplest and most satisfying exercise option. Kathy Smith's *Walkfit for a Better Body*, written by Kathy Smith, with Susanna Levin (Warner Books, 1994), can help you get started and stay motivated. It also provides a lot of supplementary information on eating, upper-body strengthening (which walking doesn't provide), proper clothing, and walking during pregnancy. Kathy Smith is one of my favorite video instructors, and this book reinforces my admiration for her work. Check http://www.Collage Video.com (see above) for her many exercise videos.

For the fainter of heart, or as a foul-weather alternative, you might also want to check out Leslie Sansome's line of indoor walking (in place) videos. This is a great option if your indoor space is limited.

Another choice well-adapted to limited space is Mindy Mylrea's gliding discs, which provide excellent low-impact cardio conditioning by allowing your foot to slide across the floor, with your heel serving as the brake. If you've tried these discs at the gym, be aware that the discs sold for home use are different—more like Frisbees than potholders, and intended for carpeted surfaces. For some reason, the gliding-disc people want to limit the availability of the potholder-type discs designed for hard surfaces to fitness professionals, though I was able to get a pair by calling (800) 464-7309. The gliding-disc videos work with either product.

The Strong Women series by Dr. Miriam Nelson of Tufts University (*Strong Women Stay Slim, Strong Women Stay Young,* and many others) is a terrific resource for anyone interested in a "civilized" strength-training program that's easily performed at home. You can purchase books at http://www.StrongWomen.com, or order from http://www.amazon.com or your local bookstore. To order the video, call (800) 203-5585. The online catalog, http://www.aswechange.com, sells the *Strong Women Stay Young* video as well as the "heavy hands" and ankle weights needed to carry out the program.

Curves, Contours Express, and Lady of America are examples of a different kind of fitness center—circuit training (short intervals of aerobic exercise alternating with intervals of strength training) with no men and no mirrors. At Curves, for example, directed by music and taped instruction, you move through eight to twelve hydraulic resistance machines that target specific body parts. The pace is intended keep your heart rate at 60 percent of maximum, verified by regular pulse taking. If you feel self-conscious about exercising in a standard gym, this approach may be just the thing for you. To find out if there's a franchise for any of these programs near your home, check your Yellow Pages or go to http://www.curvesinternational.com (for Curves), http://www.contoursexpress.com (for Contours Express), and http://www.ladiesworkoutexpress.com (for Lady of America).

Want something a little more offbeat? Guess what—the hula hoop is making a comeback. ("Grass skirt, meet the sweatsuit," wrote Jennifer Medina in the *New York Times*.) If you live in a metropolitan area, you may be able to track down a hula-hoop class. You can buy a hoop for home use at http://www.sports-hoop.com, a website that helps you choose the right hoop for your height, weight, and level of experience.

Newsflash: "Current pools" aren't just for physical therapy. If your town doesn't already have one, lobby for one at your local recreation center or fitness club. They're great for low-impact exercise as you walk or swim against the flow.

Nia, short for Neuromuscular Integrative Action, is a fusion fitness technique that blends moves from dance and martial arts in a sort of free-form program that claims to use "whole-body, grounded movement, rather than repetitive jogging or lifting." "Nia is to exercise what holistic medicine is to health care. Nia is movement as medicine." You won't find their videos or DVDs at Collage Video, so if you're interested in learning more or ordering products, visit http://www.nia-nia.com.

For something that's really fun, try Zumba. Zumba, which means "party," is based on Latin dance. As with many exercise programs, the advanced moves aren't easy, particularly for people who didn't grow up chachacha-ing, but just about anyone can manage the beginner level and take it from there. Like Nia, Zumba products aren't available at Collage Video. Their own website is http://www.zumba.com/us.

If you'd like an exercycle but don't want to pay the big bucks, you can buy a product that allows you to convert your bicycle into a stationary bike. Two setups that I have seen online are the Minoura Mag series and the Blackburn Trakstand. Prices start at around $100 and go up, depending on the features you desire.

Good deals await you if you're among the 30 percent of beginning exercisers who are still at it after nine months. Used treadmills and other exercise machinery frequently show up at neighborhood yard sales or on Craigslist. If walking or running without leaving home appeals to you, well, then, someone else's loss of motivation may be your gain!

A much cheaper exercise aid is a pedometer. K-Mart (http://www.kmart.com) sells nearly two dozen models, ranging in price from under $10 to about $25. Some of them talk to you. You can find models with built-in calorie counters, heart-rate monitors, or FM radios.

For a list of online fitness sites, check out: http://www.fitness.net top20.com.

Some women find it helpful to hire a personal trainer who can tailor a fitness program to their particular needs. Many personal trainers will provide nutritional advice as well. Good sources of referrals include your city or county recreation department, your local YMCA, private exercise clubs, or a local college with an exercise science or kinesiology department. Or try Craigslist, under Services. Factors to consider when choosing a trainer, in addition to cost, include usual clientele (athletes? fitness buffs? sedentary types? disabled or injured?), place of work (at home? at your house? inside or outside?), and policy regarding cancellations. No licensing is required for personal trainers, but you should find out whether the person you're considering has been certified by the American Council on Exercise (ACE), the Aerobics and Fitness Association of America (AFAA), or some other reputable certifying body. Ater all, you're depending on her (or him) not only to help you buff up but also to protect you from injury. Then, when you interview candidates, ask yourself if there's a good match of personalities: Do you need a drill sergeant to keep you motivated, or do you prefer someone more soft-spoken? Try to find one who gives a pretest and then does follow-up testing so you can track your progress.

Gaining a Little Weight and Still Looking Great (Chapter 5 Resources)

Regarding dressing slim: If you want something more serious and focused than *What Not to Wear* (by Trinny Woodall and her colleagues, Riverhead Books, 2003), lists of tips can be found at many websites, including: http://www.womenfitness.net/beauty/makeup/dressing.htm.

A more extended discussion of dressing slim can be found in *Does This Make Me Look Fat?* by Leah Feldon (Villard Books, 2003). Feldon is also the author of several other books on dressing and personal style.

For a book on dressing specifically aimed at "mature" women—if you can stand the annoying proliferation of typefaces—take a look at *40 Over 40: 40 Things Every Woman over 40 Needs to Know About Getting Dressed,* by Brenda Kinsel (Wildcat Canyon Press, 2000).

Also, for the slightly longer of tooth—I include myself in their numbers—is Charla Krupp's *How Not to Look Old: Fast and Effortless Ways to Look 10 Years Younger, 10 Pounds Lighter, 10 Times Better* (Springboard Press, 2008). This book is a remarkable compendium of nondietary, nonexercise, and, for the most part, nonsurgical strategies for looking Y&H ("young and hip"). Each chapter addresses a single problem area, with solutions grouped into high-, medium-, and low-maintenance approaches and ending with Krupp's personal list of "Brilliant Buys."

Special Concerns (Chapter 6 Resources)

Relationship Issues

A book that addresses relationship problems focused on food is entitled, appropriately, *Your Diet Is Driving Me Crazy,* by Cynthia Sass and Denise Maher (Marlowe & Company, 2004). To help couples who engage in "food fights," the authors present the SANITY model, an acronym for "See the problem"; "Ask your partner to understand the problem"; "Negotiate a compromise"; "Imagine creative solutions"; "Take advantage of outside resources"; and "Yuck it up…to dissolve tension." It does not specifically address dietary adjustments to smoking cessation, but the general principles can be adapted if both partners are approaching the situation with goodwill.

Pregnancy and Postpartum

A number of sites aimed at pregnant women address weight issues extensively but only incidentally deal with smoking. An online daily planner, http://www.babyfit.com offers personalized nutrition and fitness programs based on information you provide. Membership costs $19.95/year. A general pregnancy site that at least pays lip service to the need to quit smoking can be found at http://www.baby center.com/expert/pregnancy/pregquitsmoking/1405530.html.

Obesity and Large Weight Gain

"With obesity much on Americans' minds," writes Gina Kolata in the *New York Times* (1/4/05), "an entire industry has sprung up selling diets and diet books, meal replacements and exercise programs, nutritional supplements and Internet-based coaching, all in an effort to help people lose weight." No wonder we're confused! Unfortunately, almost no controlled studies have been conducted to evaluate the claims of these products and services. An exception is Weight Watchers; a controlled study published in 2003 showed a modest but real difference in outcome for Weight Watchers participants versus a randomly assigned comparison group that received no intervention but tried to lose weight on their own. This does not mean that other (perhaps less-expensive) approaches don't work; it just means that they haven't been tested. Visit http://www.weightwatchers.com to find meetings in your area or online help. Weight Watchers also offers a software program for Palm-based PDAs called On-the-Go.

Eating Disorders

Need help in finding a psychiatrist or psychologist? (A psychiatrist holds an MD degree and can prescribe medication. A psychologist is a PhD and may specialize in a variety of techniques; the cognitive behavioral approach is generally favored for eating disorders. Your best choice may depend more on the particular clinician and specialty than on the degree.) For information on finding a board-certified psychiatrist in your area, go to http://www.abpn.com/public.htm. To locate a local screening site, visit http://www.mentalhealthscreening. org. For help in finding a qualified psychologist in your area, go to http://locator.apahelpcenter.org.

For women with a history of disordered eating or severe dieting, *Intuitive Eating: A Revolutionary Program That Works* (St. Martin's Griffin, 2003) and an earlier companion volume, *Intuitive Eating: A Recovery Book for the Chronic Dieter; Rediscover the Pleasures of Eating and Rebuild Your Body Image* (St. Martin's Griffin, 1996), both by Evelyn Tribole and Elyse Resch, are highly recommended. These books feature a nondieting approach that can sustain you on the journey back to normal eating.

Depression

As noted above, under Eating Disorders, you can find information on locating a board-certified psychiatrist by going to http://www.abpn.com/public.htm. To locate a local screening site, visit http://www.mentalhealthscreening.org. For help in finding a qualified psychologist in your area, go to http://locator.apahelpcenter.org.

If you suffer from seasonal depression and want to try phototherapy, a company named Northern Light Technologies (http://www.northernlighttechnologies.com) specializes in products to meet your needs. First Street (click on http://www.firststreetonline.com) carries a line of lamps called Balanced Spectrum. Think of them as "grow lights" for people!

For more information about seasonal depression, take a look at *Positive Options for Seasonal Affective Disorder (SAD)*, by Fiona Marshall and Peter Cheevers (Hunter House, 2003), a useful compendium of information on the biological basis of SAD as well as on alternatives for treatment.

Selected Bibliography

This bibliography is not intended to be exhaustive. Rather, it provides support for the major points in each chapter and a jumping-off place for the reader who wishes to dig a little deeper. If my own articles seem disproportionately represented, it is not because I claim ownership of the entire field but because these studies form the scientific basis for much of the advice I offer in this book.

Chapter 1: What Every Woman Who Ever Smoked Should Know

Anda, R. F., D. F. Williamson, L. G. Escobedo, E. E. Mast, G. A. Giovino, and P. L. Remington. "Depression and the Dynamics of Smoking: A National Perspective." *Journal of the American Medical Association* 264 (1990): 1541–45.

Antell, D. E. "Zest England: The Top Seven Threats to Your Skin." http://www.antell-md.com/zest.html (accessed August 25, 2009).

Antell, D. E, and E. M. Taczanowski. "How Environment and Lifestyle Choices Influence the Aging Process." *Annals of Plastic Surgery* 43 (1999): 585–88.

Berlin, I., S. Said, O. Spreux-Varoquaux, R. Olivares, J. M. Launay, and A. J. Puech. "Monoamine Oxidase A and B Activities in Heavy Smokers." *Biological Psychiatry* 38 (1995): 756–61.

Califano, J. A. "The Wrong Way to Stay Slim." *NEJM* 333 (1995): 1214–16.

Clark, M. M., R. D. Hurt, I. T. Croghan, C. A. Patten, P. Novotny, J. A. Sloan, S. R. Dakhil, G. A. Croghan, E. J. Wos, K. M. Rowland, A. Bernath, R. F. Morton, S. P. Thomas, L. K. Tschetter, S. Garneau, P. J. Stella, L. P. Ebbert, D. B. Wender, and C. L. Loprinzi. "The Prevalence of Weight Concerns in a Smoking Abstinence Clinical Trial." *Addictive Behaviors* 31 (2006): 1144–52.

Copeland, A. L., P. D. Martin, P. J. Geiselman, C. J. Rash, and D. E. Kendzor. "Predictors of Pretreatment Attrition from Smoking Cessation among Pre- and Postmenopausal, Weight-concerned Women." *Eating Behaviors* 7 (2006): 243–51.

Ernster, V. J., D. Grady, R. Miike, D. Black, J. Selby, and K. Kerlikowske. "Facial Wrinkling in Men and Women, by Smoking Status." *American Journal of Public Health* 85 (1995): 78–82.

Female First. "Susan Sarandon's Advice on How Staying Looking Young" [sic]. http://www.femalefirst.co.uk/celebrity/Susan+Sarandon-1200.html (accessed August 25, 2009).

Glassman, A. H. "Cigarette Smoking: Implications for Psychiatric Illness." *American Journal of Psychiatry* 150 (1993): 546–53.

Johnson, G. K., and M. Hill. "Cigarette Smoking and the Periodontal Patient." *Journal of Periodontology* 75 (2004): 196–209.

Johnston, L. D., P. M. O'Malley, J. G. Bachman, and J. E. Schulenberg, (December 11, 2008). "More Good News on Teen Smoking: Rates At or Near Record Lows." University of Michigan News Service: Ann Arbor, MI. http://www.monitoringthefuture.org (accessed August 23, 2009).

Kluger, R. *Ashes to Ashes: America's Hundred Year Cigarette War, the Public Health, and the Unabashed Triumph of Philip Morris.* New York: Alfred A. Knopf, 1996.

Mosley, J. G., and A. C. Gibbs. "Premature Grey Hair and Hair Loss among Smokers: A New Opportunity for Health Education?" *British Medical Journal* 313 (1996): 1616.

Murphy, C. H., and P. C. Doyle. "The Effects of Cigarette Smoking on Voice-Fundamental Frequency." *Otolaryngology—Head and Neck Surgery* 97 (1987): 376–80.

Namenek Brouwer, R. J., and C. S. Pomerleau. "'Pre-quit Attrition' among Weight-concerned Women Smokers." *Eating Behaviors* 1 (2000): 145–51.

Pomerleau, C. S., A. N. Zucker, and A. J. Stewart. "Characterizing Concerns about Postcessation Weight Gain: Results from a National Survey of Women Smokers." *Nicotine & Tobacco Research* 3 (2001): 55–64.

Pomerleau, C. S., A. N. Zucker, R. J. Namenek Brouwer, O. F. Pomerleau, and A. J. Stewart. "Race Differences in Weight Concerns among Women Smokers: Results from Two Independent Samples." *Addictive Behaviors* 26 (2001): 651–63.

Striegel-Moore, R. H., D. E. Wilfley, K. M. Pike, F. A. Dohm, and C. G. Fairburn. "Recurrent Binge Eating in Black-American Women." *Archives of Family Medicine* 9 (2000): 83–87.

Trüeb, R. M. "Aging of Hair." *Journal of Cosmetic Dermatology* 4 (2005): 60–72.

U.S. Department of Health and Human Services. *Women and Smoking: A Report of the Surgeon General*. Rockville, MD: Public Health Service, Office of the Surgeon General, 2001.

Chapter 2: Managing Your Weight and Looking Great: Making Friends with Mother Nature

Chiolero, A., D. Faeh, F. Paccaud, and J. Cornuz. "Consequences of Smoking for Body Weight, Body Fat Distribution, and Insulin Resistance." *American Journal of Clinical Nutrition* 87 (2008): 801–09.

Eisenberg, D., and B. C. Quinn. "Estimating the Effect of Smoking Cessation on Weight Gain: An Instrumental Variable Approach." *Health Services Research* 41 (2006): 2255–66.

Hatsukami, D., L. LaBounty, J. Hughes, and D. Laine. "Effects of Tobacco Abstinence on Food Intake among Cigarette Smokers." *Health Psychology* 12 (1993): 499–502.

Leischow, S. J., and M. L. Stitzer. "Effects of Smoking Cessation on Caloric Intake and Weight Gain in an Inpatient Unit." *Psychopharmacology (Berl.)* 104 (1991): 522–26.

Lerman, C., W. Berrettini, A. Pinto, F. Patterson, S. Crystal-Mansour, E. P. Wileyto, S. L. Restine, D. G. Leonard, P. G. Shields, and L. H. Epstein. "Changes in Food Reward Following Smoking Cessation: A Pharmacogenetic Investigation." *Psychopharmacology (Berl).* 174 (2004): 571–77.

Lissner, L., C. Bengtsson, L. Lapidus, and C. Bjorkelund. "Smoking Initiation and Cessation in Relation to Body Fat Distribution Based on Data from a Study of Swedish Women." *American Journal of Public Health* 82 (1992): 273–75.

Klimek, V., M. Y. Zhu, G. Dilley, L. Konick, J. C. Overholser, H. Y. Meltzer, W. L. May, C. A. Stockmeier, and G. A. Ordway. "Effects of Long-term Cigarette Smoking on the Human Locus Coeruleus." *Archives of General Psychiatry* 58 (2001): 821–27.

Pinto, B. M., B. Borrelli, T. K. King, B. C. Bock, M. M. Clark, M. Roberts, and B. H. Marcus. "Weight Control Smoking among Sedentary Women." *Addictive Behaviors* 24 (1999): 75–86.

Pomerleau, C. S., E. Ehrlich J. C. Tate, J. L. Marks, K. A. Flessland,

and O. F. Pomerleau. "The Female Weight-control Smoker: A Profile." *Journal of Substance Abuse* 5 (1993): 391–400.

Pomerleau, C. S., O. F. Pomerleau,, R. J. Namenek, and A. M. Mehringer. "Short-term Weight Gain in Abstaining Women Smokers." *Journal of Substance Abuse Treatment* 18 (2000): 339–42.

Tizabi, Y., D. H. Overstreet, A. H. Rezvani, V. A. Louis, E. Clark Jr., D. S. Janowsky, and M. A. Kling. "Antidepressant Effects of Nicotine in an Animal Model of Depression." *Psychopharmacology (Berl.)* 142 (1999): 193–99.

Williamson, D. F., J. Madans, R. F. Anda, J. C. Kleinman, G. A. Giovino, and T. Byers. "Smoking Cessation and Severity of Weight Gain in a National Cohort." *New England Journal of Medicine* 324 (1991): 739–45.

Chapter 3: Eating Less and Enjoying It More

Cheskin, L. J., J. M. Hess, J. Henningfield, and D. A. Gorelick. "Calorie Restriction Increases Cigarette Use in Adult Smokers." *Psychopharmacology (Berl.)* 179 (2005): 430–36.

Guiliano, M. *French Women Don't Get Fat*. New York: Knopf, 2005.

Mehringer, A. M., C. S. Pomerleau, S. M. Snedecor, and R. Finkenauer. "Favorite Cigarette of the Day in a Random Sample of Women Smokers." *Addictive Behaviors* 33 (2008): 848–52.

Natural Resources Defense Council. "Endocrine Disruptors." http://www.nrdc.org/health/effects/qendoc.asp (accessed August 25, 2009).

Pomerleau, C.S. "Cofactors for Smoking and Evolutionary Psychobiology." *Addiction* 92 (1997): 397–408.

Rozin, P., K. Kabnick, E. Pete, C. Fischler, and C. Shields. "The Ecology of Eating: Smaller Portion Sizes in France than in the United States Help to Explain the French Paradox." *Psychological Science* 14 (2003): 450–54.

WebMD. "The Many Benefits of Breakfast." http://www.webmd.com/diet/features/many-benefits-breakfast (accessed August 25, 2009).

Chapter 4: Exercise—Minimizing Gain with Minimal Pain

American College of Sports Medicine. "ACSM Position Stand on the Recommended Quantity and Quality of Exercise for Developing and Maintaining Cardiorespiratory and Muscular Fitness, and

Flexibility in Adults." *Medicine & Science in Sports & Exercise* 30 (1998): 975–91.

Bock, B. C., B. H. Marcus, T. K. King, B. Borrelli, and M. R. Roberts. "Exercise Effects on Withdrawal and Mood among Women Attempting Smoking Cessation." *Addictive Behaviors* 24 (1999): 399–410.

Borg, G. *Perceived Exertion and Pain Scales*. Champaign, IL: Human Kinetics Publishers, 1998.

Hansen, C. J., L. C. Stevens, and J. R. Coast. "Exercise Duration and Mood State: How Much is Enough to Feel Better?" *Health Psychology* 20 (2001): 267–75.

Hu, F. B., T. Y. Li, G. A. Colditz, W. C. Willett, and J. E. Manson. "Television Watching and Other Sedentary Behaviors in Relation to Risk of Obesity and Type 2 Diabetes Mellitus in Women." *Journal of the American Medical Association* 289 (2003): 1785–91.

Jakicic, J. M., B. H. Marcus, K. I. Gallagher, M. Napolitano, and W. Lang. "Effect of Exercise Duration and Intensity on Weight Loss in Overweight, Sedentary Women: A Randomized Trial." *Journal of the American Medical Association* 290 (2003): 1323–30.

Pomerleau, M. [no relation to the author], P. Imbeault, T. Parker, and E. Doucet. "Effects of Exercise Intensity on Food Intake and Appetite in Women." *American Journal of Clinical Nutrition* 80 (2004): 1230–36.

Schneider, K. L., B. Spring, and S. L. Pagoto. "Affective Benefits of Exercise while Quitting Smoking: Influence of Smoking-specific Weight Concern." *Psychology of Addictive Behaviors* 21 (2007): 255–60.

Taylor, A., and M. Katomeri. "Walking Reduces Cue-elicited Cigarette Cravings and Withdrawal Symptoms, and Delays Ad Libitum Smoking." *Nicotine and Tobacco Research* 11 (2007): 1183–90.

U.S. Department of Health and Human Services. "2008 Physical Activity Guidelines for Americans." http://www.health.gov/PA Guidelines (accessed August 25, 2009).

Rigotti, N. A. "Treatment Options for the Weight-Conscious Smoker." *Archives of Internal Medicine* 159 (1999): 1169–71.

Ussher, M., P. Nunziata, M. Cropley, and R. West. "Effect of a Short Bout of Exercise on Tobacco Withdrawal Symptoms and Desire to Smoke." *Psychopharmacology (Berl.)* 158 (2001): 66–72.

WebMD. "What's the Best Time to Exercise?" http://www.webmd
.com/fitness-exercise/features/whats-the-best-time-to-exercise
(accessed August 25, 2009).

Chapter 5: Gaining a Little and Getting Okay with It

Linde, J. A., R. W. Jeffery, S. A. French, N. P. Pronk, and R. G. Boyle.
"Self-weighing in Weight Gain Prevention and Weight Loss
Trials." *Annals of Behavioral Medicine* 30 (2005): 210–16.

Perkins, K. A., M. Levine, M. Marcus, S. Shiffman, D. D'Amico,
A. Miller, A. Keins, J. Ashcom, and M. Broge. "Tobacco Withdrawal in Women and Menstrual Cycle Phase." *Journal of Consulting and Clinical Psychology* 68 (2000): 176–80.

Perkins, K. A., M. D. Marcus, M. D. Levine, D. D'Amico, A. Miller,
M. Broge, J. Ashcom, and S. Shiffman. "Cognitive-behavioral
Therapy to Reduce Weight Gain Concerns Improves Smoking
Cessation Outcome in Weight-concerned Women." *Journal of
Consulting and Clinical Psychology* 69 (2001): 604–13.

Pomerleau, C. S., A. W. Garcia, O. F. Pomerleau, and O. G. Cameron.
"The Effects of Menstrual Phase and Nicotine Withdrawal on
Nicotine Intake and on Biochemical and Subjective Measures in
Women Smokers: A Preliminary Report." *Psychoneuroendocrinol-
ogy* 17 (1992): 627–38.

Pomerleau, C. S., and C. L. Kurth. "Willingness of Female Smokers
to Tolerate Postcessation Weight Gain." *Journal of Substance Abuse*
8 (1996): 371–78.

Van Cauter, E., and K. L. Knutson. "Sleep and the Epidemic of Obesity in Children and Adults." *European Journal of Endocrinology*
159 Suppl 1 (2008): S59–66.

Chapter 6: Special Concerns
Relationship Issues

Andrews, G. "Intimate Sabateurs." *Obesity Surgery* 7 (1997): 445–48.

Ball, K., and D. Crawford. "An Investigation of Psychological, Social
and Environmental Correlates of Obesity and Weight Gain in
Young Women." *International Journal of Obesity* 30 (2006):
1240–49.

Jong-Fast, M. (1998). "A World Apart." *Mode.* (*Mode* is no longer
published, but the article can be viewed at http://www.ericajong
.com/old_site/mjfmode9805.htm.) (accessed August 25, 2009).

Russ, C. S., P. A. Ciavarella, and R. L. Atkinson. "A Comprehensive Outpatient Weight Reduction Program: Dietary Patterns, Psychological Considerations, and Treatment Principles." *Journal of the American Dietetic Association* 83 (1984): 444–46.

Pregnancy and Postpartum

Abraham, S., W. King, and D. Llewellyn-Jones. "Attitudes to Body Weight, Weight Gain, and Eating Behavior in Pregnancy." *Journal of Psychosomatic Obstetrics & Gynecology* 15 (1994): 189–95.

Berg, C. H., E. R. Park, Y. Chang, and N. A. Rigotti. "Is Concern about Post-cessation Weight Gain a Barrier to Smoking Cessation among Pregnant Women?" *Nicotine & Tobacco Research* 10 (2008): 1159–63.

Levine, M. D., M. D. Marcus, M. A. Kalarchian, L. Weissfeld, and L. Qin. "Weight Concerns Affect Motivation to Remain Abstinent from Smoking Postpartum." *Annals of Behavioral Medicine* 32 (2006): 147–53.

Park, E.T., Y. Chang, V. Quinn, S. Regan, L. Cohen, A. Viguera, C. Psaros, K. Ross, and M. Rigotti. "The Association of Depressive, Anxiety, and Stress Symptoms and Postpartum Relapse to Smoking: A Longitudinal Study." *Nicotine and Tobacco Research* 11 (2009): 707–14.

Pomerleau, C. S., R. J. Namenek Brouwer, and L. T. Jones. "Weight Concerns in Women Smokers During Pregnancy and Postpartum." *Addictive Behaviors* 25 (2000): 759–67.

Obesity

Flegal, K. M., B. I. Graubard, D. F. Williamson, and M. H. Gail. "Excess Deaths Associated with Underweight, Overweight, and Obesity." *Journal of the American Medical Association* 394 (2005): 1861–67.

Han, T. S., F. C. Bijnen, M. E. Lean, and J. C. Seidell. "Separate Associations of Waist and Hip Circumference with Lifestyle Factors." *International Journal of Epidemiology* 27 (1998): 422–30.

National Heart Lung and Blood Institute. "Aim for a Healthy Weight." http://www.nhlbi.nih.gov/health/public/heart/obesity/lose_wt/index.htm (accessed August 25, 2009).

Large Weight Gain

National Heart Lung and Blood Institute, "Aim for a Healthy Weight." http://www.nhlbi.nih.gov/health/public/heart/obesity/lose_wt/index.htm (accessed August 25, 2009).

Williamson, D. F., J. Madans, R. F. Anda, J. C. Kleinman, G. A. Giovino, and T. Byers. "Smoking Cessation and Severity of Weight Gain in a National Cohort." *New England Journal of Medicine* 324 (1991): 739–45.

Disordered Eating

American Psychiatric Association. *Diagnostic and Statistical Manual of Mental Disorders, 4th ed.* (DSM-IV). Washington DC: American Psychiatric Association, 1994.

Bulik, C. M., R. E. Dahl, L. H. Epstein, and W. H. Kaye. "The Effects of Smoking Deprivation on Caloric Intake in Women with Bulimia Nervosa." *International Journal of Eating Disorders* 10 (1991): 451–59.

Frank, R. E., M. K. Serdula, and D. Adame. "Weight Loss and Bulimic Eating Behavior: Changing Patterns within a Population of Young Adult Women." *Southern Medical Journal* 84 (1991): 457–60.

Kendzor, D. E., C. E. Adams, D. W. Stewart, L. E. Baillie, and A. L. Copeland. "Cigarette Smoking Is Associated with Body Shape Concerns and Bulimia Symptoms among Young Adult Females." *Eating Behaviors* 10 (2009): 56–58.

King, T. R., M. Matacin, B. H. Marcus, B. C. Bock, and J. Tripolone. "Body Image Evaluations in Women Smokers." *Addictive Behaviors* 25 (2000): 613–18.

Krahn, D. D., C. L. Kurth, M. Demitrack, and A. Drewnowski. "The Relationship of Dieting Severity and Bulimic Behaviors to Alcohol and Other Drug Use in Young Women." *Journal of Substance Abuse* 4 (1992): 341–353.

Pomerleau, C. S., E. Ehrlich, J. C. Tate, J. L. Marks, K. A. Flessland, and O. F. Pomerleau. "The Female Weight-control Smoker: A Profile." *Journal of Substance Abuse* 5 (1993): 391–400.

Pomerleau, C. S., and D. Krahn. "Smoking and Eating Disorders: A Connection?" *Journal of Addictive Diseases* 12 (1993): 169.

Pomerleau, C. S., and K. K. Saules. "Body Image, Body Satisfaction, and Eating Patterns in Normal-weight and Overweight/Obese Women Current Smokers and Neversmokers." *Addictive Behaviors* 32 (2007): 2329–34.

Pomerleau, C. S., A. N. Zucker, and A. J. Stewart. "Characterizing Concerns about Postcessation Weight Gain: Results from a National Survey of Women Smokers." *Nicotine & Tobacco Research* 3 (2001): 55–64.

Welch, S. L., and C. G. Fairburn. "Smoking and Bulimia Nervosa." *International Journal of Eating Disorders* 23 (1998): 322–27.

Depression

American Psychiatric Association. *Diagnostic and Statistical Manual of Mental Disorders, 4th ed.* (DSM-IV). Washington DC: American Psychiatric Association, 1994.

Covey, L. S., A. H. Glassman, and F. Stetner. "Depression and Depressive Symptoms in Smoking Cessation." *Comprehensive Psychiatry* 31 (1990): 350–54.

Dunn, A. L., M. H. Trivedi, J. B. Kampert, and C. G. Clark. "Exercise Treatment for Depression." *American Journal of Preventive Medicine* 28 (2005): 1–8.

Frank, E. *Gender and Its Effects on Psychopathology.* Washington, DC: American Psychiatric Press, 2000.

Glassman, A. H. "Cigarette Smoking: Implications for Psychiatric Illness." *American Journal of Psychiatry* 150 (1993): 546–53.

Goel, N., M. Terman, J. S. Terman, M. M. Macchi, and J. W. Stewart. "Controlled Trial of Bright Light and Negative Air Ions for Chronic Depression." *Psychological Medicine* 35 (2005): 945–55.

Heatherton, T. F,. L. T. Kozlowski, R. C. Frecker, and K. O. Fagerström. "The Fagerström Test for Nicotine Dependence: A Revision of the Fagerström Tolerance Questionnaire." *British Journal of Addiction* 86 (1991): 1119–27.

Heatherton, T. F., L. T. Kozlowski, R. C. Frecker, W. Rickert, and J. Robinson. "Measuring the Heaviness of Smoking: Using Self-reported Time to the First Cigarette of the Day and Number of Cigarettes Smoked Per Day." *British Journal of Addiction* 84 (1989): 791–99.

Lasser, K., J. W. Boyd, S. Woolhandler, D. U. Himmelstein, D. Mc-Cormick, and D. H. Bor. "Smoking and Mental Illness: A Population-based Prevalence Study." *Journal of the American Medical Association* 284 (2000): 2606–10.

Niaura, R., D. M. Britt, W. G. Shadel, M. Goldstein, D. Abrams, and R. Brown. "Symptoms of Depression and Survival Experience among Three Samples of Smokers Trying to Quit." *Psychology of Addictive Behaviors* 15 (2001): 13–17.

Odendaal, J. S. J., and R. A. Meintjes. "Neurophysiological Correlates of Affiliative Behaviour Between Humans and Dogs." *The Veterinary Journal* 3 (2003): 296–301.

Oren, D. A., K. L. Wisner, M. Spinelli, C. N. Epperson, K. S. Peindl, J. S. Terman, and M. Terman. "An Open Trial of Morning Light Therapy for Treatment of Antepartum Depression." *American Journal of Psychiatry* 159 (2002): 666–69.

Pomerleau, C. S., J. L. Marks, and O. F. Pomerleau. "Who Gets What Symptom? Effects of Psychiatric Cofactors and Nicotine Dependence on Patterns of Nicotine Withdrawal Symptomatology." *Nicotine and Tobacco Research* 2 (2000): 275–80.

Pomerleau, C. S., R. J. Namenek Brouwer, and O. F. Pomerleau. "Emergence of Depression During Early Abstinence in Depressed and Non-depressed Women Smokers." *Journal of Addictive Diseases* 20 (2001): 73–80.

Chapter 7: Quitting for Good

Abrams, D. B., R. Niaura, R. A. Brown, K. M. Emmons, M. G. Goldstein, and P. M. Monti. *The Tobacco Dependence Treatment Handbook: A Guide to Best Practices.* New York: Guilford Press, 2003.

American Psychiatric Association. *Diagnostic and Statistical Manual of Mental Disorders, 4th ed.* (DSM-IV). Washington, DC: American Psychiatric Association, 1994.

DiFranza, J. R., J. A. Savageau, K. Fletcher, J. K. Ockene, N. A. Rigotti, A. D. McNeill, M. Coleman, and C. Wood. "Recollections and Repercussions of the First Inhaled Cigarette." *Addictive Behaviors* 29 (2004): 261–72.

Fiore, M. C., C. R. Jaén, T. B. Baker, et al. *Treating Tobacco Use and Dependence: 2008 Update.* Clinical Practice Guideline. Rockville, MD: Public Health Service, US Department of Health and Human

Services. http://www.ncbi.nlm.nih.gov/books/bv.fcgi?rid=hstat2
.chapter.28163 (accessed August 25, 2009).

Gallagher, J. *The Dialogue: An International Journal of Faith, Thought, and Action.* "Linda Hyder Ferry: Dialogue with a Physician for Such a Time as This." http://dialogue.adventist.org/articles/10 _3_gallagher_e.htm (accessed August 25, 2009).

National Institutes of Health. National Institute on Drug Addiction. "Research Report Series—Tobacco Addiction." http://www.drug abuse.gov/researchreports/nicotine/nicotine.html (accessed August 25, 2009).

Noble, H. B. (2 March 1999) *The New York Times* "New from the Smoking War: Success." http://www.nytimes.com/1999/03/02/ science/new-from-the-smoking-wars-success.html?scp=1&sq= linda%20ferry&st=cse (accessed August 25, 2009).

Patterson, F., C. Jepson, A. A. Strasser, J. Loughead, K. A. Perkins, R. C. Gur, J. M. Frey, S. Siegel, and C. Lerman. "Varenicline Improves Mood and Cognition During Smoking Abstinence." *Biological Psychiatry* 65 (2009): 144–49.

Pomerleau, O. F., C. S. Pomerleau, and R. J. Namenek. "Early Experiences with Nicotine among Women Smokers, Ex-smokers, and Never-smokers." *Addiction* 93 (1998): 595–99.

Pomerleau, C. S., O. F. Pomerleau, R. J. Namenek, and J. L. Marks. "Initial Exposure to Nicotine in College-age Women Smokers and Never-smokers: A Replication and Extension." *Journal of Addictive Diseases* 18 (1999): 13–19.

Schnoll, R. A., F. Patterson, and C. Lerman. "Treating Tobacco Dependence in Women." *Journal of Women's Health* 16 (2007): 1211–18.

Sherva, R., K. Wilhelmsen, C. S. Pomerleau, S. A. Chasse, J. P. Rice, S. M. Snedecor, L. J. Bierut, R. J. Neuman, and O. F. Pomerleau. "Association of a SNP in Neuronal Acetylcholine Receptor Subunit Alpha 5 (CHRNA5) with Positive Experience ('Pleasurable Buzz') during Initial Smoking." *Addiction* 103 (2008): 1544–52.

U.S. Department of Health and Human Services. "FDA: Boxed Warning on Serious Mental Health Events to be Required for Chantix and Zyban." http://www.fda.gov/NewsEvents/Newsroom /PressAnnouncements/ucm170100.htm (accessed August 25, 2009).

Chapter 8: The Chic of Quitting

American Heart Association. "Women and Cardiovascular Disease Facts." http://www.americanheart.org/presenter.jhtml?identifier= 3039318 (accessed August 25, 2009).

Centers for Disease Control and Prevention. *2004 Surgeon General's Report—The Health Consequences of Smoking.* http://www.cdc.gov/ tobacco/data_statistics/sgr/2004/index.htm (accessed August 25, 2009).

Centers for Disease Control and Prevention. "Smoking and Tobacco Use—Health Effects." http://www.cdc.gov/tobacco/basic_informa tion/health_effects/index.htm (accessed August 25, 2009).

Shea, A. K., and M. Steiner. "Cigarette Smoking During Pregnancy." *Nicotine and Tobacco Research* 10 (2006): 267–78.

U.S. Department of Health and Human Services. *The Health Benefits of Smoking Cessation.* Public Health Service, Centers for Disease Control. Center for Chronic Disease Prevention and Health Promotion, Office on Smoking and Health, Rockville, MD, 1990.

U.S. Department of Health and Human Services. *Women and Smoking: A Report of the Surgeon General.* Public Health Service, Office of the Surgeon General; Rockville, MD, 2001.

Index

About the Author

Cynthia S. Pomerleau has had a varied career characterized by a long-standing interest in women's issues. She wrote her doctoral dissertation on autobiographies of English women in the seventeenth and eighteenth centuries at the University of Pennsylvania and subsequently directed an Oral History Project on Women Physicians at the Medical College of Pennsylvania. Working in a medical school library piqued her interest in health research and led her to return to school for training in psychology and neuroscience.

From 1985 until her retirement in 2009, she worked in the University of Michigan Department of Psychiatry as a research professor and as director of the Nicotine Research Laboratory, where much of her research focused on the impact of smoking on women (e.g., menstrual cycle effects, postcessation weight gain, depression). She is the author of more than a hundred articles and book chapters on smoking and a contributor to the *2001 Surgeon General's Report on Women and Smoking*. She continues her active involvement in writing and scientific investigation as research professor emerita.

She lives in Ann Arbor and Empire, Michigan, with her husband and collaborator, Ovide Pomerleau, and their two cats, Tabasco and Marshmallow. They also have two grown daughters, Julie and Aimée, a son-in-law, Jeff, and two grandchildren, Augie and Claudia.